Table of Contents

Introduction 4

Chapter 1: What Is the Ketogenic Diet? The Science Behind It 6

How Ketosis Works 6

The Balance of Ketosis 7

Make A Keto Plan...7

Elements of Ketosis 9

The Biology – How it Works 9

Chapter 2: The Benefits & Downsides of Keto 14

The Benefits of The Ketogenic Diet 14

The Downsides Of The Ketogenic Diet..............................16

Chapter 3: Keto Versus Other Diet Plans 19

Chapter 4: The Ketogenic Diet for Weight Loss......21

Chapter 5: Foods to Eat and Ones to Avoid 24

Best Foods & Drinks for Ketosis.................................24

The Right Snack Foods – Grab & Go 39

Foods and Beverages to Avoid While in Ketosis..................44

Chapter 6: How to Go "Keto" 46

How to Get Started 46

Get Down to The Basics...47

Chapter 7: How to Know If You Are in Ketosis 63

Chapter 8: Diet & Exercise: The Right Combination 66

Provide the Balance 66

A Beginner Regimen for Your Exercise Plan......................67

Super Tips for Keto and Your Exercise Routine 69

The Stalling and Plateaus of Weight Loss 77

Chapter 9: Ketogenic Diet FAQs 79

Chapter 10: Living the Keto Lifestyle....................82

Preparing Keto Meals on A Budget 82

Measure Your Food with Accuracy 84

Use the Slow Cooker..85

Dining Out Tips 87
Common Mistakes Using the Keto Diet.................88

Chapter 11: Ketogenic Recipes **91**

11.1: Breakfast Recipes 91

Bacon – Spinach - Avocado & Egg 91
Baked Eggs in Avocado 93
BLT Breakfast Salad...94
Brussels Sprouts, Eggs & Bacon for Brunch.......96
Cheesy Egg & Spinach Nest 98
Cheesy Muffins...100
Coconut Flour – Cream Cheese Pancakes 102
Kale – Avocado & Egg Skillet...........................104
Perfect Scrambled Eggs 106

11.2. Beverages 107

Bulletproof Coffee 107

11.3. Bread...108

Keto Bread..108
90-Second Bread-In-A-Mug............................110

11.4. Lunchtime Delights 111

Alfredo Pizza..111
Bacon Stir Fry for Brunch................................113
Broccoli & Cheese Soup 114
Carnitas - Crockpot...116
Crockpot Chicken Chowder 118
Cucumber Sandwich 120
Pizza Bites 121

11.5. Salads 122

Chicken Salad 122
Chopped Greek Salad.....................................124
Salmon & Caesar Salad...................................125
Shrimp & Avocado Salad 127
Tomato – Avocado & Cucumber Salad 129

11.6. Dinner Specialties...................................130

Beef Short Ribs..130

Buffalo Chicken Casserole 132
Bun-less Bacon Burgers 134
Cheesy Steak 135
Chuck Steak – Slow Cooker 137
Coconut Shrimp 138
Feta-Stuffed Burgers 139
Fried Pork Chops 141
Garlic Parmesan Wings 142
Meatballs in the Crock 143
Pork Kabobs 145
Steak Pinwheels 147

11.7. Side Dishes 149

Baked Radishes & Brown Butter Sauce 149
Baked Zucchini Gratin 151
Buttery Mushrooms - Slow Cooked 153
Cauliflower 'Potato' Salad - Vegetarian 154
Parmesan & Pork Rind Green Beans 156
Vegetarian Deviled Eggs 157

11.8. Desserts 159

Chocolate Avocado Pudding 159
Chocolate Mousse 160
Chocolate Shakes 161
Crustless Cheesecake Bites 162
Lemon Blueberry Muffins 163
Lemonade Fat Bombs 165
NY Cheesecake Cupcakes 167
Peanut Butter & Chocolate Cups 169
Raspberry Fudge 171

11.9. Appetizers & Snacks 173

Cheese Chips & Guacamole 173
Chicken-Pecan Salad & Cucumber Bites 175
Crunchy Zucchini Sticks 177
Smoked Salmon & Cream Cheese Roll-Ups 179

Chapter 12: Your 14-Day Meal Plan 181
Conclusion 187

Introduction

I am so excited that you have chosen to take a new path using the Ketogenic diet plan using your personal copy of the *Ketogenic Diet: The Complete Guide to Healthy Weight Loss*. Thank you for doing so. Before you begin your life-changing dieting methods, let's view some of the history involved around the keto type of eating.

During the Paleolithic Period, humans were known to hunt for their protein and gather their vegetables, fruits, nuts, and seeds to survive. Because this method isn't ideal in today's society; you don't have to search for food each day. That was the way people lived centuries ago which made the body develop a survival mechanism to survive during times when food was scarce.

Whenever a person encountered satiation where they consumed more calories than they burned, the unused calories would be converted into fat fuels and stored for emergency starvation times. This mechanism was useful in times where nutrient resources were scarce and required a lot more energy to locate.

However, in modern times, food is not only natural to come by, but most meals that are affordable are packed full of unnecessary calories. Our bodies continue to create these fat stores, even though the times of hunting and gathering are behind us. These facts were taken into consideration when the ketogenic diet was developed.

The only way to lose fat is to trick the body into burning it. If you specifically consume meals high in fats and very low-lacking in carbohydrates; your body will believe that the only fuel available is fat. It will then enter what is known as ketosis, which is a process whereby the liver releases more ketones. Ketones form as a result of burning fats for fuels.

Starvation mode is known when the body is calories deficient and lacking in the nutrients it needs. Many people have forced their bodies into starvation mode in a desperate attempt to lose weight. However, what few people realize, is that the weight loss while in starvation mode is usually muscle tissue. The body holds onto its emergency fat stores until the last possible moment. Ketosis is a form of starvation mode that takes this fact away. You won't be depriving your body of calories, or nutrients. You will be starving your body of carbohydrates and sugars. Consider using intermittent fasting techniques which will be discussed later on.

The following chapters will provide you with some of the detailed guidelines for the keto dieting method from the beginning. You will also be provided with many delicious recipes for lunch, dinner, or just any time of the day that you are hungry.

Let's start with the science behind the Ketogenic Diet.

Chapter 1: What Is the Ketogenic Diet? The Science Behind It

With the high-fat and low-carb traits, the keto diet is similar to the Atkins Diet and other low-carb diets. The process drastically reduces your intake of carbohydrates to replace it with fat. This loss places the body into a state of ketosis – a metabolic state. Many things begin to happen as you burn the
fat for energy. You are burning fat into ketones in your liver to
supply energy for your brain.

How Ketosis Works

A ketogenic diet will help you reduce your calorie intake to below the volume of calories your body can use up daily. It is essential to beckon the energy stockpiled in the fat cells to deliver fuel or energy to your muscles.

The keto diet will limit the volume of carbs you consume. A substantial percentage of your fuel for the day will come from fat transformed to ketones. Once you have the protein, carbohydrates, and fat ratio monitored by the diet plan such as shown in this book; you are well on the way to a successful diet strategy.

You will not be over-eating with large portions of protein. You won't eliminate fat or carbs which make it a useful and safe diet plan for fat loss. If you take the approach of eating less, without considering your diet—you will be losing essential minerals and vitamins you need daily—which can result in muscle spasms, fatigue, mental fogginess, hunger, headaches, irritability, insomnia, and emotional depression. You can also lose valuable muscle mass; not just the pounds you intended to drop.

By using the lower carb keto plan, you can reduce your carbohydrates, calorie counts, and nurture your body with the suitable amount of water, meat, eggs, fish, veggies, nuts, as well as high-quality oils which create fat loss minus the unpleasant side effects.

The Balance of Ketosis

Before you get started, you should understand how the nutrients work using the ketogenic diet plan. The macronutrients are building blocks of food consisting of protein, fat, and carbs.

This is just an Example: In general, for a regular American diet, you will have a diet plan that is generally composed of 16% protein, 34% of calories from fat, and approximately 50% of the calories from carbs. The ketogenic technique mixes it up with 15-20% protein, 70-75% fat, and 5-15% from carbohydrates. Of course, as you will learn, these totals are guidelines and not 'set-in-stone.'

Everyone's totals are different since your percentages are calculated according to your weight, age, gender, body fat percentage, and activity levels. You can go online and type in *Ruled Me* or other sites and use the keywords '*keto macro calculator*' to locate the scale guideline. Just type in your information, and it will provide you with your macro limits.

Track the macros, either by hand or by the use of apps such as Spark People or My Fitness Pal. This is the most accurate way to ensure you are remaining in ketosis and have no danger of over-eating. Use any method that works for you. Once you have the numbers, you are ready to go.

Make A Keto Plan

According to a favorite dieting resource, your focus is to intake between 20 to 35 grams of *net* carbohydrates daily. Of course, if you can maintain your diet plan to 20 grams of *net* carbs, you will lose the weight quicker. (You are ahead of the game plan since all of the recipes have totals calculated + the meal plan.) These are the four plans to consider before you begin your diet plan:

- *Ketogenic Technique # 1*: The standard ketogenic diet (SKD) consists of moderate protein, high-fat, and is low in carbs. This particular technique has approximately 5% carbs, 75% fats, and 20% proteins.

- *Ketogenic Technique # 2*: The targeted keto diet (TKD), will provide you with a technique to add carbs to the diet plan during the times when you are working out.

- *Ketogenic Technique # 3*: The cyclical ketogenic diet (CKD) is observed with five-keto days followed by two high-carbohydrate days. You can also be a full week using the keto diet followed by 1 higher carbohydrate day.

- *Ketogenic Technique # 4*: The high-protein keto diet is comparable to the standard keto plan (SKD) in all aspects. However, it does have more protein.

These four plans make dieting an excellent choice for all of your needs. The first plan is the one most commonly used.

Count Those Carbs

Before you are entirely in gear, you need to start carb counting to make sure you keep your body in perfect 'sync' with the plan. Reading the labels may be a bit nerve-racking in the beginning, but after a while, it will be like you have always done it that way.

Remember this Formula: Total Carbs minus (-) Fiber = Net Carbs. The good part is that each of the recipes in this book already has the total net carbs calculated for you. Just eat and enjoy!

Elements of Ketosis

If you don't consume enough carbs from your food; your cells will begin to burn fat for the necessary energy instead. Your body will switch over to ketosis for its energy source as your cut back on your calories and carbs.

Two elements that occur when your body doesn't need the glucose:

- The Stage of Lipogenesis: If there is a sufficient supply of glycogen in your liver and muscles, any excess is converted to fat and stored.

- The Stage of Glycogenesis: The excess of glucose converts to glycogen and is stored in the muscles and liver. Research indicates that only about half of your energy used daily can be saved as glycogen.

Your body will have no more food (similar to when you are sleeping) making your body burn the fat to create ketones. Once the ketones break down the fats, which generate fatty acids, they will burn-off in the liver through beta-oxidation. Thus, when you no longer have a supply of glycogen or glucose, ketosis begins and will use the consumed/stored fat as energy.

The Biology – How it Works

To know how the keto diet works, it helps to have a basic understanding of how your body uses food for energy. It's a complicated process which has remained distinctly unchanged throughout the years. Let's start by differentiating between atoms and molecules.

Atoms are the smallest identifiable units of an element. The combination of protons, neutrons, and electrons defines the atom's physical and nuclear properties. Think of atoms as individual parts used to build a house – that is, nails, insulation, boards and such. Each one is physical and has properties that are distinct from each other, but *all* are necessary for a substantial house.

Molecules are composed of two or more atoms. Despite this, molecules do not represent the nature of the atoms they are composed of. For example, Na (sodium) is a silvery metal that reacts violently with water. As in it goes 'boom.' On the opposite side of the Periodic table, we have Cl, chlorine, which can cause fatal damage to your respiratory system. When combined, the sodium ion and chlorine anion form table salt, NaCl.

And lastly, table salt doesn't explode or cause your lungs to blister until you drown in your own blood. Sure, table salt is dangerous in too high a quantity, but the amount people usually consume it, salt is harmless. The point being is that atoms and molecules are very different. Think of molecules as parts to a house, such as a wall or a frame for a window. It is only one part of a much larger structure but is made of smaller, physically distinct components.

In biology, there are four types of large biological molecules, called LBMs for short. These molecules consist of carbohydrates, lipids, proteins, and nucleic acids. Each has unique roles in how your body works, and without any one of them, we wouldn't be able to live.

Monomers are single units of a molecule. When monomers of the same type of molecule chain together, they form polymers. The exception to this rule is lipids, which are not polymers as they can consist of many different molecules.

In general terms, these four classes of molecules don't exist outside of non-living things.

With molecules, structure implies function. That is, the shape of the molecule defines what your body does with it. Painkillers work as they fit in neural pathways like jigsaw pieces. Doing this blocks the paths that register pain, in simple terms.

All molecules, regardless of function or shape, store energy – the potential to do work. There are two energy classifications; kinetic energy (in motion) and potential energy (at rest).

Potential energy rests in the bonds between atoms and molecules. Pretend potential energy is gasoline in a car. It is inert, at rest. Breaking those bonds releases that energy into a system, enabling it to function. To use the car analogy, igniting the gasoline releases heat and force, causing the engine to run.

It is important to remember that energy cannot be created or destroyed. That's the first law of thermodynamics. Energy can only transfer between systems. The expansion of gases in the combustion chamber of your car moves the piston, which results in your car moving. The potential energy of the gasoline 'becomes' the kinetic energy of your car moving.

For your benefit, we will ignore proteins and nucleic acids. We will deal instead with the first two classes of LBM: carbohydrates and lipids.

Carbohydrates

Glucose, $C_6H_{12}O_6$, is a carbohydrate molecule which our bodies use as a source of energy. This is true for all animals. You might know it as sugar or 'simple' sugar. It consists of 12 hydrogen atoms, six carbon atoms, and six oxygen atoms.

Lipids

The most critical lipid is fat. That's what you're worried about, isn't it? You don't want that fat piling on, that's why you bought this book. Before we shy away from fat, it's important to remember that fat is a vital component of a healthy body. Too much or too little fat are both dangerous. Your body needs some fat to remain healthy.

Fat, like sugar - and plenty of other molecules - stores potential energy. But in our 'sugar-saturated' lives, our bodies don't use fat for your energy the same way it uses carbohydrates – that is, sugars, for energy.

But now that I've mentioned it – how does your body get energy from carbs?

Carbohydrates Metabolism

Metabolism is the sum of all chemical reactions taking place in your body. It is necessary for you to function. Some of us have 'high' metabolism, and some of us don't. Sometimes our metabolism slows as we age.

As mentioned, our world is saturated with carbohydrates, it's not like you can just turn a key and get the energy you need. Humans must process them first.

Once you ingest foods, your stomach breaks these carbohydrates down into smaller monomers like glucose. The glucose is distributed throughout your body where it is stored in cells. These cells use the glucose – and oxygen that you've breathed in, as fuel. They then release water and carbon dioxide as waste products.

But what if your body can't get the carbohydrates it needs? You know, for example, when you're on a keto diet? That energy must come from somewhere else.

Remember those ketone bodies we talked about earlier; acetone, acetoacetic acid, and all that? Your liver produces these during periods of fasting – or low carb intake, or starvation. These ketone bodies are distributed, like carbs, about your body and absorbed into cells, which use them for energy. This is a state called ketosis. Don't confuse this with ketoacidosis.

In ketosis, your body metabolizes fat at a higher rate than it would otherwise. And that is, of course, the reason keto can work for you.

Fats Metabolism

Remember the ketone bodies discussed earlier. These are: acetone, acetoacetic acid, etc. Your liver produces these ketones during periods of fasting, low carbohydrate intake or starvation. These ketone bodies are distributed, like carbohydrates, over your body and are absorbed into the cells, which use them for energy. When this occurs at higher levels and becomes the most used way to obtain energy in our body, instead of glucose, the state of ketosis is reached. Ketosis should not be confused with ketoacidosis, which refers to an excessively high number of ketones in our body that can be counterproductive.

In ketosis the body metabolizes fat more quickly than it would in a different state. This is the reason why ketosis is ideal for burning fat and losing weight quickly as well as healthy.

Chapter 2: The Benefits & Downsides of Keto

As with any diet, there are advantages and disadvantages. The ketogenic diet is not any different. However, it is well known because it does work for weight loss. Why not improve your health at the same time? Some of the issues you encounter can be remedied. Those improvements will be shown in this segment.

The Benefits of The Ketogenic Diet

Metabolic Syndrome: This is a collection of syndromes grouped together which enhances the risk of heart disease and diabetes. These include high blood pressure, high blood sugar, low HDL cholesterol, abdominal obesity, and high levels of triglycerides.

Lower Blood Pressure: The ketogenic low-carb diet is an excellent way to lower your blood pressure. It is advisable to speak with your physician about reducing your meds while on the plan. If you begin to feel dizzy; that is one of the first signs the lack of carbs is working. You are headed in the right direction.

Pre-diabetes and Diabetes: Excess fat may be effectively removed with the keto plan which is what is linked to pre-diabetes, type-2 diabetes, and metabolic syndrome. One of the first studies was performed in 2005 at Duke University, North Carolina.

The study researched 28 overweight participants who had type 2 diabetes. The trial was performed for 16 weeks. During the study, the patients consumed less than 20 grams of carbs daily – while at the same time lowering the diabetic medications. Overall, the final results revealed the patients could reduce or discontinue the medications. For the most beneficial outcomes, it is important to seek a doctor's advice for these options.

Improvement of Your Cholesterol Profile: An arterial buildup is generally associated with the triglyceride and cholesterol levels, which have been proven to improve with the keto diet plan.

Obesity & Overweight Individuals: Many individuals exceed what is considered healthy figures when it comes to weight. It is imperative to use the keto diet plan to get started on the right path for weight loss.

Improved Thinking Skills: Your brain is approximately 60% fat by weight. Therefore, you might become confused as you consume high-fat foods. By increasing your fatty foods intake; you will have better chances to better your mind. It can maintain itself and work at full capacity.

Acne Relief: By eating fewer processed foods and less sugar; your insulin levels will be lowered, and the acne should improve.

Alzheimer's Disease Improved: The disease's progression can be slowed and the symptoms reduced with the keto plan.

Cancer Treatments: Several types of cancer and slow tumor growths are being treated using the keto diet.

Epilepsy Treatments: Reductions from seizures have occurred in children who use the ketogenic diet.

Polycystic Ovary Syndrome (PCOS): This is the utmost endocrine disorder affecting young women of child-bearing years and is also associated with insulin resistance, obesity, and hyperinsulinemia. According to the *US National Library of Medicine - The National Institutes of Health, better known as NCBI*; a 6-month study concluded a significant improvement in weight and fasting women over a 24-week period. The group limited carb intake to 20 grams daily for the 24 weeks.

Gum Disease and Tooth Decay Remedied: The pH balance in your mouth is influenced by sugar intake. Your gum issues could subside after about three months on a keto diet plan. You will be consuming healthier foods.

Lack of Hunger: The enormous benefit occurs because fat is naturally more satisfying than just carbs. You just need to wait a little longer to become satiated after a meal. The high-fats will cause the full-state to last longer.

Important Note: Seek your doctor's advice before changing your eating patterns. In some cases, you could reduce the need for some medications.

You are now ready to begin your new way of living a healthier life. Follow the simple guidelines, and you will start to burn the fat!

The Downsides Of The Ketogenic Diet

These are some of the most common problems you will face when you change over to the keto diet plan:

Thirst is Increased: Fluid retention is increased when you are consuming carbohydrates. Once the carbs are flushed away, water weight is lost. You counter-balance by increasing your water intake since you are probably dehydrated during the first week or so of the diet switch.

In a conventional diet, if you're dehydrated your body can use the stored carbs to restore hydration. When you're in ketosis, the carbs are removed, and your body doesn't have the water reserves.

If you have tried other diets, you might have been dehydrated, but the higher carbohydrate counts stopped you from being thirsty. Thus, the keto state is a diuretic state.

Bad Breath Becomes Evident: Some new dieters might experience what is described as a nail polish odor to other people or a fruity aroma. This is a ketone body known as acetone. It may also be displayed as a body odor with the changes occurring. Be sure to maintain good oral health and use a breath freshener when needed.

Take into account that diet soda and chewing gum are not generally allowed on the keto diet because they reduce ketones. Therefore, only use it temporarily. If you are at home, just grab the toothbrush.

Pungent Urine Smells Are Present*:* With the high acetone levels, your urine is also a strong clue to ketosis (its darkened color). There is no reason for concern; it's just your body adjusting to the new status.

Constipation Issues: Dehydration can be a factor on a low-carbohydrate diet such as the keto plan. You should add a bit of salt to your food and consume plenty of water. Eating the right veggies will also help with the movements. Milk of Magnesia may be the answer to your tummy issues.

Induction Flu Issues: This is a stage where you feel lethargic, a bit confused, irritable, nauseated, and have a headache. Within several days the symptoms will typically withdraw. Try adding ½ teaspoon of salt to a glass of water and drink it. This may take fifteen or twenty minutes to be effective. You may also repeat the mixture daily for the first week if you are queasy.

Leg Cramps: The loss of magnesium (a mineral) can be a demon and create pain with the onset of the keto diet plan changes. With the loss of the minerals during urination, you could experience attacks of cramps in your legs.

Heart Palpitations: You may begin to feel 'fluttery' as a result of dehydration or because of an insufficient intake of salt. Try to adjust your menu plan by trying more carbs, but if you don't feel better quickly, you should seek emergency care.

Disruptive Sleep Patterns: Some dieters experience a pattern of waking up during the night—too restless to sleep. This may be caused by low serotonin and insulin levels. Try a square of chocolate (70% if possible), and ½ of a tablespoon of fruit spread. Vitamin supplements have also been reported to cause sleeping issues if taken at night.

Chapter 3: Keto Versus Other Diet Plans

According to Women's Health Magazine, the Atkins, Ketogenic, and Dukan diet are all the craze since each one limits carbohydrate intake. However, there are some differences to consider.

How Ketogenic Compares to Low-Carb - Atkins and Paleo Plans

The Keto Diet limits the carbohydrate intake at 5% of the energy intake whereas the low-carb diet plans have no definition. The ketogenic diet is moderate protein, high-fat, and low-carbs. With its limitations of carbs, the diet plan forces your body to burn the fat for energy (ketosis).

The Atkins Plan: You have four phases of the plan and don't have to count the calories but must count the carbs. During the introductory stage, the Atkins diet is set at roughly 15-30 grams per day of carbs to help promote fat burning instead of using glycogen for energy. Its popularity took a dive when individuals were gaining weight over the long term, getting sick, and increasing their blood lipid profile.

The Paleo diet is a newer trend based on eating as our ancestors did 10,000 years ago. It consists of eating more fruits and veggies because meat supplies were not always available daily. The foods contain more fiber, omega-3s, vitamins, and minerals. They also had less salt and saturated fats. Fats aside from meat should come from healthy oils (avocado, macadamia, walnut, olive). The balance of the diet should reflect refined sugar, legumes, potatoes, cereal grains, and dairy.

The Dukan diet also consists of four phases; two for losing weight, and two for maintaining. The process becomes a bit hectic as each phase moves to the next.

Keto Wins

Unlike the Dukan Diet and Atkins plan, you don't need to work the diet plan in phases. Instead, you just follow your high-protein, high-fat, and low-carbohydrate routine until you reach your desired weight. You don't have to continue with a maintenance program. You just keep eating the delicious meals such as the ones provided in this book. The debate continues, because not everyone believes Keto is the way, but many do!

Go for the win and combine the ketogenic diet with an exercise plan, you will discover long-term success. Enjoy the delicious meals, snacks, and desserts and find new ways of creating energy. Up the fat while lowering the carbs is a 'win-win' combination. Next, you will learn which foods you will be enjoying while taking the ketosis journey.

Chapter 4: The Ketogenic Diet for Weight Loss

The dieting techniques used on the keto diet are effective for weight loss when you get all of the components working together.

Protein & Its Importance

Protein is a must for your dieting plan for these reasons:

Muscle Repair and Growth: Protein should be increased on days you are more active. It's essential to have an idea and understand the balance of carbs, proteins, and fats. The balance is the goal you are attempting to achieve, and it's found in a focused plan such as the keto diet.

Protein Saves Your Calories: Protein slows down your digestion process making you feel more satisfied with the foods you consume. During the first segment of your diet plan, it's imperative that you feel full, so there's no temptation to cheat with your menu selection.

Protein is a Fat Burner: Science has proven your body can't use and burn your fat as quickly as energy sources produce - unless you have help from either carbs or protein. The balance of protein must be maintained to preserve your calorie-burning lean muscles.

How Your Carbohydrate Intake Is Balanced

Your body exchanges 100% of the carbs of your intake and turns it into glucose which gives your body an energy boost. About 50%-60% of your intake of calories is produced by those carbs which are stored in your liver as glycogen and is released as your body needs it.

Glucose is essential for the creation of adenosine triphosphate (ATP) which is an energy molecule. The fuel from glucose is vital for the daily maintenance and activities inside your body. After the liver has reached its maximum capacity for its limits, the excessive carbohydrates turn into fat.

In most cases, the following guidelines will be useful for you. Research has indicated the process is successful in approximately 90% of cases. Since there's no set rule for carb intake, you will want to be sure you are consuming the right amounts of food to keep your diet balanced for ketosis.

You will be gradually working your way through the plan considering these food options by consuming plenty of vegetables, a minimal intake of carbs and two to three pieces of fruit daily.

- Daily Intake of 0-20 Grams of Net Carbs: You will discover most of the foods in this meal plan are dedicated to 20 or just above 20 grams daily.

- Moderate Net Carbs – 20-50 Net Carbs Daily: If you are obese, have diabetes, or metabolically deranged, this is the plan for you. If you are consuming less than the 50 grams daily; your body will achieve a ketosis state which supplies the ketone bodies. Be sure you eat plenty of low-carb veggies. Have some berries with whipped cream. You can also enjoy avocado, nuts, and seeds that only have a few trace carbons.

- Moderate or Liberal Intake Amounting To 100-150 Grams Daily: If you are active and lean trying to maintain weight, enjoy several fruits daily. Consider eating all of the veggies you can eat.

The Difference Between a Low-Carb & Ketogenic Diet Plan

Don't get a low-carb diet confused with a keto diet. A low-carb diet will average 200 (+) carbs and can charge you up to 100 grams daily. Your long-term effect of a low-carb diet plan may differ substantially depending on the number of fats and proteins that are consumed. Each of the recipes in this book is ketogenic.

Chapter 5: Foods to Eat and Ones to Avoid

Choosing free-range/organic food items when possible - is foremost when it is time to start your new techniques for meal preparation. If you are pressed for time, it's vital for you to have access to delicious and nutritious food. As a guideline consider adjusting your diet to some of the healthier food items as shown in this book.

It is essential to understand which fats are dangerous and which ones are good for your health. You must make a balance between the Omega-6s and the Omega-3s. Tuna, trout, shellfish, and salmon are a beneficial choice for the balance of Omega-3.

It is advisable to choose raw and organic milk products. You can also use full-fat products over low-fat or fat-free products.

Flours used from seeds and nuts are excellent substitutes for regular flour which can include almond flour and milled flax seeds. Macadamias, almonds, and walnuts are also a good choice if eaten in small amounts.

Best Foods & Drinks for Ketosis

Stock the Pantry

You want your ingredients to be keto-friendly Begin with these items:

- Coconut flour
- Quinoa
- Splenda & Stevia
- Sugar-free ketchup
- Sugar-free gelatin

- Unsweetened cocoa powder
- Yellow mustard
- Pickles (limit sweet or bread & butter)
- Natural nut butter – no sugar

Legumes

Many legumes are off-limits on the keto plan, however, in small amounts, you can enjoy green beans and peas.

Preferred Spices

You will need to become a label reader for spices because many of the pre-made products contain sugar. Use these items:

- Sea Salt
- Black Pepper – White Pepper
- Cinnamon
- Basil
- Cayenne Pepper
- Chili Powder
- Cilantro
- Italian seasoning

Stock the Refrigerator

It is essential to maintain your health using dairy products. It is best to choose fresh, raw or organic milk products. It is also vital to purchase full-fat dairy items. The harder cheeses usually have fewer carbs. You can also add additional protein and calcium using non-dairy products such as cashew or almond milk.

These are a few of the products and the categories where they qualify:

- Sour cream

- Soft and hard cheeses (for example sharp cheddar, or mozzarella)
- Almond, Cashew, or coconut milk
- Cottage cheese
- Heavy whipping cream
- Kefir
- Cream cheese
- Sour cream
- Parmesan cheese
- Ghee – also called clarified butter
- Grass-Fed Butter: You can promote fat loss and is almost carb-free. The butter is a naturally occurring fatty acid which is rich in conjugated linoleic acid (CLA). It is suitable for maintaining weight loss and retaining lean muscle mass.

Stock Up on Healthy Protein Products

The keto plan focuses on quality proteins, not carbohydrates. You will see many items listed as a starting point for your snacks.

- Whole Eggs: Search for a local area market for free-range options. You can scramble, fry, boil, or devil eggs up for a picnic or any occasion.

- Fish: Go back to nature because it is preferable to eat any foods that are caught in the wild. Include tuna (fresh & canned), trout, salmon, snapper, eel, catfish, flounder, cod, halibut, mahi-mahi, or mackerel as part of your diet plan – portioned in bags to freeze

- Shellfish: Choose crabs, clams, lobster, oysters, scallops, squid, shrimp, or mussels.

- Pastured Pork & Poultry: Choose from duck, chicken, pheasant, or quail.

- Turkey: Breasts & ground turkey

- Chicken: Thighs, breasts, drumsticks, & ground chicken

- Meat: Grass-fed is preferred because it has a better fatty acid count. Choose from lamb, veal, goat, or other wild game. Cuts of beef include flank steak, sirloin, chuck roast, lean ground beef, etc.

- Venison: This is an excellent choice since it is lean, as well as vegetarian-raised meat.

- Fresh nuts: Almonds, Hazelnuts, Macadamia, Pecans, Pine nuts, Cashews, Walnuts, Pistachios, etc.

- Fresh Seeds: Sesame seeds, flax seeds, chia seeds, Psyllium, etc.

- Peanut Butter: Try natural peanut butter but use caution because they do contain high counts of carbohydrates and Omega-6s. Macadamia nut butter is a wise alternative.

Purchase Healthy Fats

To achieve success in the ketogenic diet, you need fats, but remember not all fats are created equal. This is the 'low-down' facts on fats:

The Good Fats

- **Monounsaturated Fats: Avocados**: Purchase this healthy food which has 24 grams-30 grams of healthy fats and is also high in fiber. Also included are extra-virgin olive oil (EVOO) and avocado oil.

- **Saturated Fats:** This is found in palm or coconut oil (MCTs), cream, eggs, lard, ghee, butter, and red meat.

- **Natural Trans Fats**: Found in meat and dairy products from grass-fed animals

- **Natural Polyunsaturated Fats**: Omega-3 is found in fish oil, fish, chia, and flaxseeds. Note: For legumes, seeds, and nuts rich in Omega-6 but just eat in small portions. The ratio of Omega-3 compared to Omega-6 should be as close as possible of 1:1.

These are a few more examples of good fat items:
- Flaxseed oil
- Olives: You can use olives in many recipes and salads with its high fiber and fat counts.

The Bad Fats

You need to be aware of the ones that fall into this category:

- **Processed Trans Fats**: Avoid fast foods, processed foods, margarine, and commercially prepared baked goods.

- **Processed Polyunsaturated Fats**: Avoid these oils: Sunflower, peanut, grapeseed, sesame, corn, canola, and soybean.

Purchase Your Vegetables

You can enjoy veggies any time of day. Each of these has the Net Carbs listed per 100 grams or 1/2 cup:

- Alfalfa Seeds – Sprouted - 0.2 g
- Arugula – 2.05 g
- Asparagus – 1.78 g

- Bamboo shoots: 3 g
- Beans – Green snap – 3.6 g
- Beet greens – 0.63 g
- Bell pepper – 4.6 g
- Broccoli – 4.04 g
- Broccoli raab – 0.15 g
- Cabbage – savoy – 3 g
- Carrots – 6.78 g
- Carrots – baby – 5.34 g
- Cauliflower – 2.97 g
- Celery – 1.37 g
- Chard – 2.14 g
- Chicory greens – 0.7 g
- Chives – 1.85 g
- Coriander – Cilantro Leaves – 0.87 g
- Cucumber with Peel – 3.13 g
- Eggplant – 2.88 g
- Garlic – 30.96 g
- Ginger root – 15.77 g
- Kale – 5.15 g
- Leeks – bulb (+) lower leaf – 12.35 g
- Lemongrass – citronella 25.31 g
- Lettuce – red leaf – 1.36 g
- Lettuce – crisp-head types ex. iceberg 1.77 g
- Mushrooms brown – 3.7 g
- Mustard Greens – 1.47 g
- Onions – yellow – 7.64 g
- Onions – scallions or spring – 4.74 g
- Onions – sweet – 6.65 g
- Peppers – banana – 1.95 g
- Peppers – red hot chili – 7.31 g
- Peppers – jalapeno – 3.7 g
- Peppers – sweet – green – 2.94 g
- Peppers – sweet – red – 3.93 g
- Peppers – sweet – yellow – 5.42 g
- Portabella Mushrooms – 2.57 g

- Pumpkin – 6 g
- Radishes – 1.8 g
- Seaweed – kelp – 8.27 g
- Seaweed – spirulina - 2.02 g
- Shiitake mushrooms – 4.29 g
- Spinach – 1.43 g
- Squash o crookneck, summer – 2.64 g
- Squash - Zucchini – 2.11 g
- Squash – winter – acorn – 8.92 g
- Tomatoes – 2.69 g
- Turnips – 4.63 g
- Turnip Greens – 3.93 g
- White Mushrooms – 2.26 g

Special Notes:

- Kale: Your heart health can be significantly improved with the rich nutrients including magnesium and folate.

Purchase Your Fruits

This collection of keto fruits will offer you under 7 grams of net carbs per 1/2 cup or 100 grams:

- Green olives
- Avocados
- Coconut
- Rhubarb
- Black Olives
- Carambola aka Starfruit
- Lemon juice
- Lime juice
- Strawberries
- Casaba Melon
- Gooseberries
- Prickly pears

- Acerola, aka West Indian Cherry
- Oheloberries
- Boysenberries
- Grapefruit

Consider raspberries; many of the professionals believe this is one of the healthiest and most nutritious fruits. A 1/2 cup serving merely carries 5.4 net carbs as well as many health-protective polyphenols which help fight oxidative stress. A handful is enjoyable with a splash of heavy cream.

What about blackberries? This is a delicious 5 net carbs for a 1/2 cup serving. Add some heavy cream.

Your Best Beverages

The best guideline is to keep it simple and drink plenty of water. You can also flavor your drinks using stevia-based flavorings or lemon juice. Consider some of these drink choices. This chart is calculated with your grams of carbs derived for you:

- Water: 0 g
- Water with lemon: 0 g
- Tea: 0 g – 1 sugar cube = 4 g
- Coffee: 0 g – 1 sugar cube = 4 g
- Diet soft drink: 0 g– Beware of artificial sweeteners
- 8 oz. Almond milk, unsweetened: 2 g
- 1 cup coconut water: 9 g
- 1 cup soy milk: 12 g
- 1 cup orange juice: 26 g

A Word About Coffee & Tea: If you are struggling during your dieting plan, it is always good to know you can enjoy black coffee and unsweetened tea for -0- net carbs. Even better there is a recipe in the breakfast section of the cookbook for Bulletproof Coffee; also -0- net carbs.

Your Sweetener Choices:

You need to look at the ingredient list on the package and be sure the product doesn't have fillers such as dextrose, maltodextrin, or polydextrose which can create spikes in your blood sugar. You will also have additional carbs from the fillers.

Each of the following suggestions will be shown as the most popular to the ones that are in less demand by the majority of keto diet users. Most of your ketogenic recipes are flexible on the type of sweetener used, so it is up to you. There are a few to consider:

The #1 Choice: The best all-around sweetener is Pyure's Organic All-Purpose Blend with less of a bitter aftertaste versus a stevia-based product. The blend of stevia and erythritol is an excellent alternative to baking, sweetening desserts, and various cooking needs. The substitution ratio is one teaspoon of sugar for each one-third teaspoon of Pyure. Add slowly and adjust to your taste since you can always add a bit more.

If you need powdered sugar, just grind the sweetener in a NutriBullet or high-speed blender until it's very dry.

The #2 Choice: Swerve Granular Sweetener is also an excellent choice as a blend. It's made from non-digestible carbs sourced from starchy root veggies and select fruits. Give it a try if you don't like the taste of stevia.

Start with ¾ of a teaspoon for every one of sugar. Increase the portion to your liking. Swerve also has its own confectioners/powdered sugar for your baking needs. On the downside, it is more expensive (about twice the price) than other products such as the Pyure. You have to decide if it's worth the difference.

The #3 Choice: Xylitol is at the top of the sugary list. It is excellent for sweetening your teriyaki and BBQ sauce. It tastes just like sugar! The natural occurring sugar alcohol has the Glycemic index (GI) standing of 13. If you have tried others and weren't satisfied, this might be for you.

Xylitol is also known to keep mouth bacteria in check which goes a long way to protect your dental health. The ingredient is commonly found in chewing gum. Unfortunately, if used in large amounts, it can cause diarrhea - making chewing gum a laxative if used in large quantities.

Urgent Pet Warning: If you have a puppy in the house, be sure to use caution since it is toxic to dogs (even small amounts).

The #4 Choice: Stevia Drops are offered by *Sweet Leaf* and offer delicious flavors including hazelnut, vanilla, English toffee, and chocolate. Enjoy making a satisfying cup of sweetened coffee and drinks. Some individuals think the drops are too bitter. At first, use only three drops to equal one teaspoon of sugar.

The #5 Choice: Lakanto's Maple-Flavored Syrup is an excellent choice for pancake syrup since it is monk-fruit and erythritol based. Golden Monk Fruit Sweetener also has a brown sugar choice.

The name monk-fruit came from the Buddhist monks over 1,000 years ago and is considered a cooling agent. It may not agree with your digestive system, so use it sparingly if using in baked goods.

You will notice each of these have a GI (Glycemic Index) next to them. This is a measurement of how much your blood sugar is raised after you consume a specific food. If there is a zero (0) next to it; that means it will not increase your blood sugar counts. The measurement can reach 100 which is the baseline of insulin.

- Aspartame – GI: 0
- Erythritol - GI: 0
- Monk Fruit GI: 0
- Xylitol- GI:13
- Sucralose (liquid) GI: Variable
- Stevia (liquid) - GI: 0
- Inulin – GI: 0
- Maltitol – GI: 36
- Saccharin – GI: Variable

Alcohol Consumption Guidelines:

If you enjoy consuming alcohol, according to a favorite source, you will be glad to know you can enjoy moderate consumption. Be sure you consider the stronger liquors are posted at zero or very low in carbs. Each of the ones listed in the wine and beer section is an estimated total carb count, so you have a general idea of how many you need to adjust your daily totals.

- Vodka

- Whiskey

- Tequila

- Rum

- Scotch

- Brandy

- Cognac

- Wine – Whites – average carbs per glass

      Champagne - 1.5 g
      Chardonnay - 3.7 g
      Pinot Grigio - 3.2 g
      Riesling - 5.5 g

- Wine – Reds

Cabernet - 3.5 g
Merlot - 3.7 g
Pinot Noir - 3.4 gg

- Select Beers

    Amstel Light -5 g
    Bud Select - 3.1 g
    Coors Light - 5 g
    Michelob Ultra - 2.6 g
    Miller Lite - 3.2 g
    Rolling Rock Green Light - 2.4 g

You need to limit the intake of other alcoholic drinks which will include:

- Flavored liquor
- Cocktails
- Mixers: Soda, Juice, or Syrup

Special Note: Drink responsibly and enjoy in small amounts to prevent any health issues.

High-Carb to Low-Carb Substitutions

As you begin your new and healthier lifestyle, you will discover many shortcuts or substitutes to help you stay on track. Some of these replacements will help:

- **Flour:** Almond flour only contains 3 grams of carbs for 1/4 of a cup. Coconut flour has 6 grams, but totals are overwhelming for the regular wheat flour at 24 grams. This is why it is not on your diet plan!

- **Breadcrumbs**: You can still enjoy your crunchiness by replacing regular breadcrumbs with crushed pork rinds. The good news is that the pork rinds have zero carbs. Next time enjoy the healthier fats.

- **Tortillas**: Get ready to say no to this one which weighs in at approximately 98 grams for just 1 serving. Instead, enjoy a lettuce leaf at about 1 gram per serving. You will still have the healthy crunch!

- **Regular Rice**: Replace the standard serving portions of white or brown rice with some cauliflower rice. You can enjoy 1 cup for about 45 grams of carbs versus the 2.5 grams packed in for 1 cup of its partner.

- **Pasta**: Replace pasta using zucchini. You use a spiralizer and make long ribbons to cover your plate. It is excellent for many dishes served this way.

- **Mashed Potatoes**: Kick the regular bowls of mashed potatoes to the side and enjoy some mashed cauliflower.

You can enjoy these along with any of the regular entrees, just remember to add your carbs and enjoy.

The Condiment Issues

One huge issue that can become a problem in your state of ketosis is the condiments that are offered in most supermarkets. You are probably wondering how to prepare a keto-friendly meal. If so, this short segment is a special bonus for some of those times when nothing else will work in your particular keto recipe. Some of these will fit right in with your new batch of keto recipes.

Keep your ketosis in line with one of these favorites:

Avocado Mayonnaise

4 servings
Macronutrients: 1 g Protein | 5 g Fats | 4 g Carbs| 1 g Net Carbs

Ingredients:
- 1/2 tsp. ground cayenne pepper
- Pinch of pink salt
- Juice of 1/2 lime
- 1/2 med. avocado
- 1/4 cup olive oil

Method:
1. Dice the avocado. In a blender or food processor, combine the avocado, salt, cayenne, cilantro, and lime juice.
2. When smooth, stir in the oil – 1 tablespoon at a time - pulsing in between each addition.
3. You can store the mayo for up to one week in a sealed glass bottle.

Caesar Dressing

4 servings
Macronutrients: 2 g Protein | 23 g Fats | 2 g Carbs| 2 g Net Carbs

Ingredients:
- 1/2 cup mayonnaise
- 1 tbsp. Dijon mustard
- Juice of 1/2 lemon
- 1/2 tsp. Worcestershire sauce
- 1/4 cup parmesan cheese
- Pinch of each:
  -Freshly cracked black pepper
  -Pink Himalayan salt

Method:
1. Whisk the lemon juice, mustard, mayonnaise, salt, pepper, and Worcestershire sauce. Stir well and add the parmesan. Whisk until smooth.
2. You can store up to one week in a glass container in the fridge.

Chicken Liver Spread

1 serving
Macronutrients: 24.9 g Protein | 42.4 g Fats | 1.5 g Carbs| 1.5 g Net Carbs

Ingredients:
- 3.5 oz. chicken livers
- 1 pinch or to taste – Pepper and Salt
- 1 tsp. Italian seasoning
- 3 tbsp. softened butter

Method:
1. Add all of the fixings into a blender to form a paste.
2. Enjoy on radish slices or crackers.

Chunky Style Blue Cheese Dressing

4 servings
Macronutrients: 7 g Protein | 32 g Fats |3 g Carbs| 3 g Net Carbs

Ingredients:
- 1/2 cup of each:
  -Mayonnaise
  -Sour cream
- Juice of 1/2 lemon
- 1/2 tsp. Worcestershire sauce
- To Taste: Black pepper and salt
- 2 oz. crumbled blue cheese

Method:
1. Whisk all of the fixings except for the cheese until well mixed.
2. Fold in the cheese gently and store in a closed glass dish for up to one week.

Sriracha Mayo

4 servings
Macronutrients: 1 g Protein | 22 g Fats |2 g Carbs| 2 g Net Carbs

Ingredients:
- 2 tbsp. Sriracha sauce
- 1/4 tsp. paprika
- 1/2 cup mayonnaise
- 1/2 tsp. of each powder:
  -Onion
  -Garlic

Method:
1. Whisk the fixings together in a small container.
2. Store in an airtight glass container for up to one week in the fridge.

The Right Snack Foods – Grab & Go

Take the time to prep high-quality snacks like are provided in this cookbook. Stick to the macros including the net carbs, protein, and fat. As crazy as it sounds, you also need to consume snacks that consist of mostly fat. This makes your homemade treats an excellent choice when you are on the ketogenic diet plan. The snacks will also help you lose weight because they are balanced.

When you choose snacks, be sure to select ones that are low in carbs so your ketone levels will not be disrupted. If you have a busy lifestyle, pick some of the ones in the below list, but always remember to count the carbs. Try some of these choices the next time you don't have time to plan ahead:

- Eggs: Take a few extra minutes to prepare a batch of eggs. Prepared eggs generally store for up to a week in the fridge. It only has 0.9 grams of net carbs per egg.

It will also provide you will essential selenium, vitamin A, phosphorus, and folate.

- Avocados: This super whole food is a fantastic choice for on-the-go. Slice it into the desired portions (count the carbs) and give it a shake of pepper and salt. Try a sprinkle of grated parmesan for a taste change. You can load up on potassium and magnesium for 1.8 grams of net carbs for a 1/2 cup serving.

- Cherry Tomatoes: This is an excellent 'handful' treat but one that must be used in small amounts because the carbs do add up quickly. They reel in 2.7 carbs for a 1/2 cup portion. However, they are also a super boost of potassium, vitamin K, biotin, and vitamin C.

- Pickles: It is a great day when you can grab a pickle which is loaded with potassium and sodium to replenish your electrolytes. You can also drink the juice. For a 1 cup portion – it only contains only 1.6 net carbs.

- Olives: Watch out for additional oils added, but this is one great treat right out of the jar.

- Cucumbers: Enjoy a crispy cucumber with or without the peel. Enjoy knowing that it is an excellent source of dietary fiber as well as vitamin C and K. Enjoy 1/2 of a cup for only 1 gram of net carbs.

- Sardines: Enjoy these without guilt at zero carbs. You also get a healthy dose of fat.

- Nuts & Seeds: Create some tasty meals (in moderation) when adding seeds and nuts to your keto diet plan. Use fattier nuts including macadamias, brazil nuts, walnuts, and almonds or seeds like chia, pumpkin, and flaxseed which are high in omega 3s.

Use caution and stay away from butter that contain polyunsaturated oils/vegetable oil.

Consider this about the macadamias; they are high in a heart-healthy fat in olive oil called oleic acid. The macadamia has a crunchy taste, but on the inside, they're butter and soft – so delicious.

- String Cheese: Choose the full-fat version without additional fillers.

- A Slice of Cheese: Enjoy a slice of cheddar cheese, gouda, feta, or some parmesan. However, always check the specific type for the carbohydrate counts.

- Laughing Cow Cheese Wheels: Purchase full-fat versions and get *real* cheese when possible.

- Moon Cheese: Yes, this is real and is a crunchy cheese. It is 100% natural cheese which is similar to potato chips in cheese form.

- Beef Jerky: Watch out for the added sugars if you purchase jerky ready-made. Choose ones with only a few additional ingredients. If you enjoy preparing food, why not try making your homemade jerky. You will know for sure it's healthy!

- Seaweed Snacks: Search the labels to make sure they do not contain significant amounts of oil. Try one such as *gimMe*.

- Pork Rinds: Use these to replace chips and crackers which are a higher quality without a lot of offensive oil content. For example, try some Parmesan & Pork Rind Green Beans (see the recipe). You can also enjoy 1 14.2 gram serving of pork rinds for -o- net carbs. How does that sound?

- Pepperoni Slices: Enjoy with a high-fat cheese but keep in mind, these are highly processed. Limit the amounts used and search for hormone-free or organic if possible.

- Cacao Nibs: You can enjoy the same crunch when used as an alternative to chocolate chips.

- Quest Bars: This is an excellent travel aid, but it should be used as a last resort. Even though they are low-carbs because of the erythritol sweetener, they are processed foods you usually avoid. Just pop them into the toaster oven for a few minutes on each side.

- Nugo-Smarte Carb Bars: This is great for a treat but does contain 2 grams of carbs for each bar.

- Stevia Sweetened Dark Chocolate: If you are not using stevia, be sure it's a minimum of 80% or higher in cocoa content. Typically, the bars are about 10 carbohydrates per ounce.

- Sugar-Free Jell-O or Popsicles: You can purchase this ready-to-go or make your own.

- Iced Coffee: Leave the sugar out of your coffee and use only full-fat milk or cream. Add a bit of MCT oil powder which can be purchased as chocolate, vanilla, or unflavored.

- Greek Yogurt: The fat content is a plus for your ketogenic meal planning. Just be sure you purchase one that has no sugar added. Check each brand for the macros because each one varies. However, it is very filling, and so many are packaged in convenient smaller traveling sizes.

- Low-Carb Ice Cream: Breyers CarbSmart® gives you the opportunity to enjoy a 1/2 cup portion for only 4 net carbs. It is sweetened with erythritol.

Delicious Homemade Possibilities

These are just a few of the snacks you can prepare at home. Many of these have recipes included in this book. Just keep in mind that low-carb foods do not always mean they are keto-friendly.

Veggie Sticks with Keto-friendly Dip: This is a delicious treat using cucumbers, celery, and yellow, red, or green bell peppers. Try dipping a portion of the sticks into a specially prepared keto-friendly dip. The choices are unlimited and will vary with the net carbs (of course).

Berries with Heavy Cream: Prepare this with unsweetened – no-sugar add real heavy cream. Enjoy with your favorite berries. Be sure to count the carbs and not over-indulge.

Cinnamon Greek Yogurt & Walnuts: For only 6 grams of carbs have 2 ounces of whole milk Greek yogurt with 1/2 of a teaspoon of cinnamon, and 1 tablespoon on chopped walnuts.

Boiled Eggs: Nothing is more accessible than adding your eggs to a pot of cold water. Cover them about an inch. Use medium-high heat and let them boil. Remove from the burner and let them rest in the water 8 to 10 minutes. Drain, put in an ice bath and enjoy.

Get Your Greens: Grab 1 large collard greens leaf (no stem) and spread 1 teaspoon each of mayo and Dijon mustard. Add 1 oz. of sliced cheddar cheese and roll into a wrap (1.3 carbs).

Healthy Deli-Cut Meats & Cheese: Enjoy a simple - healthy roll-up of deli meat such as turkey breast and your favorite full-fat keto-friendly cheese.

Low-Carb Finger Food Sandwiches: Use a piece of lettuce, spinach, or slice of cheese as a sandwich in place of bread and enjoy a quick and easy egg or tuna salad.

Steak Bites: If you have a steak in the fridge that was left over from last night, cut off a few bite-sized pieces for -0- carbs (4 oz.).

Foods and Beverages to Avoid While in Ketosis

There are many healthy options to choose from while on the ketogenic diet. Avoid the foods in the following groups – unless they are structured within this cookbook or other professional sources you trust. Each food item has been calculated with all of the nutritional information listed.

Fruits: Raspberries, blueberries, and cranberries contain a high sugar content. In small portions; you can enjoy some strawberries.

Cashews and Pistachios: The high carb content should be monitored for these yummy nuts.

Artificial Sweeteners: Several types to avoid include saccharin, sucralose, and Splenda.

Regular Dairy Milk: Avoid regular dairy for sure since it packs almost 13 grams of carbohydrates per cup.

Hydrogenated Fats: Cold-pressed items should be avoided when using vegetable oils such as safflower, olive, soybean, or flax. Coronary heart disease has been linked to these fats which also include margarine.

Processed Foods: If you see carrageenan on the label, it is best to leave it on the shelf. Don't feel too guilty if you crave all of those processed foods. It happens.

As a rule of thumb, look for labels with the least amount of ingredients. Usually, the ones that provide the most nutrition are listed in those 'short' lists.

According to a popular source, here are some processed snacks to avoid while on a ketogenic diet. Some are surprising because they were deemed for years as a healthy snack. Do you recognize any of them?

- Cereal Bars
- Rice cakes
- Flavored Nuts
- Popcorn
- Potato Chips
- Pretzels
- Protein Bars
- Crackers

Beverages:

Diet Soda: Artificial sweeteners can cause you to go out of ketosis if you consume large amounts of diet drinks. Therefore, you have to use it in moderation. Research has shown a link between artificial sweeteners and sugar cravings, making it more challenging to curb those types of drink.

Chapter 6: How to Go "Keto"

Before you begin your journey to ketosis, you will need to take a few steps to get in gear with your new lifestyle changes. These suggestions will get you headed in the right path:

How to Get Started

- **Carb-Proof the Kitchen:** One of the easiest ways to stay on your plan is to remove the temptations. Remove the chocolate, candy, bread, pasta, rice, and sugary sodas you have supplied in your kitchen. If you live alone, this is an easy task. It is a bit more challenging if you have a family. The diet will also be useful for them if you plan your meals using the recipes included in this book.

- **Read Those Labels:** Almost every food item in today's grocery store has a nutrition label. Be sure you read each of the ingredients to discover any hiding carbs to keep your ketosis in line. You will be glad you took the extra time.

- **Create a Food Journal:** If you cheat, that has to count also. It will be a reminder of your indulgence, but it will help keep you in line. Others may believe you are obsessed with the plan, but it is your health and well-being that you are improving.

- **Prepare a Menu and Food Plan:** Use some of the recipes in this book and combine them with your other ketogenic favorites. You will be surprised how many tasty items you can enjoy that are full of healthy nutrients.

- **Head to the Supermarket**: When you go shopping for your ketogenic essentials be sure you take your new skills, a grocery list, and search the labels.

Get Down to The Basics

Step 1: Lower Your Carb Consumption

One of the most essential elements in achieving ketosis is a very low-carbohydrate diet. Your cells usually use the sugar/glucose as a primary fuel source, but most of your cells can also use other sources for fuel such as fatty acids as well as ketones. When the carb intake is lowered, the levels of the insulin hormone decline which allows the fatty acids to be released from fat storage in your body.

Some individuals need to limit their intake of net carbs which are your total carbs minus fiber to 20 grams daily, whereas others can remain in ketosis while eating twice that amount. If you can restrict your intake to 20 net carbs or less for the first two weeks, you will be guaranteed that ketosis is reached. At that time, you can relax and maintain the ketosis state.

Step 2: Increase the 'Healthy Fat' Intake

Consuming plenty of healthy fats can help boost your ketone levels. The lowered carbohydrate intake teams up with the high fats to produce ketosis. If you are using the ketogenic diet for weight loss, you can also achieve 60% to75% of your calories from fats. Note that the 'old-style' ketogenic diet plan as it was created for epilepsy is higher with 85% to 90% of the calories from fat.

It is essential to use high-quality food sources since you are consuming such a large percentage of your diet from fat intake. Consider using these good fats for your cooking needs; butter, coconut oil, avocado oil, and lard.

You will soon discover how many high-fat foods are low in carbs, but you still need to count them to prevent losing the ketosis state. In general, you should consume a minimum of 60% of calories from fat to boost the ketone levels. Choose from both animal and plant sources.

Step 3: Add Coconut Oil to Your Ketogenic Diet Program

The oil is also used as one of the best ways to improve ketone levels in people with nervous system disorders, such as those with Alzheimer's disease.

Coconut oil contains medium-chain triglycerides which speed up the ketosis process. Unlike many other fats, the MCTs are absorbed rapidly and go directly to the liver. There, they are castoff for immediate energy – resulting in conversion to ketones. The oil contains four types of these fats, 50% of which comes from the lauric acid.

Research has indicated the higher percentage may produce sustained ketosis levels because it is metabolized more gradual than other MCTs. Add coconut oil slowly to your diet because it can cause some stomach cramping and diarrhea until you adjust. Start the doses using one teaspoon daily and work it up to two to three tablespoons over the span of a week.

Step 4: Maintain Protein Intake

You must supply your liver with amino acids which can be used for making new glucose (gluconeogenesis). Your liver produces the glucose for the cells and organs in your body that cannot use ketones as fuel. This includes portions of the brain, kidneys, and red blood cells.

Protein also maintains muscle mass when the carb intake is lowered, especially during a weight loss program. Research has indicated the preservation of your muscle mass, and physical performance is at maximum speed when the intake range is 0.55-0.77 grams per pound of lean mass.

Think of it in simpler terms; excessive protein intake may suppress ketone production, whereas consuming too little can lead to muscle mass loss.

Step 5: Test the Ketone Levels & Make Adjustments

Your commitment is evident, but you are not sure if the keto diet is working for you. There is only one way to know for sure. You need to purchase the Ketone Test Strips (more in the next chapter) to discover your counts when you check the measurement stick against the chart on the side of the bottle.

You must keep in mind; the time of day is significant when you perform the test. Don't drink a lot of water, but don't test when you are dehydrated either. The test results won't be accurate. Be sure to follow the package instructions to the "tee" for the most informative results.

Step 6: Know What Your Body is Craving

When you live such a hurried lifestyle sometimes; you just don't know you want. Your body will tell you what is necessary to keep it going. The message is sent to you as a craving. Here are a few cravings with what your body needs and a quick fix for the issue:

- Carbs/Bread/Pasta: You need some nitrogen which can be remedied with some high protein meat.

- Chocolate: The carbon, magnesium, and chromium levels are screaming for some spinach, nuts, and seeds, or some broccoli and cheese.

- Fatty or Oily Foods: The levels of calcium and chloride need repair with some spinach, broccoli, cheese, or fish.

- Sugary Foods: Several things can trigger the desire for sugar, but typically phosphorous, and tryptophan are the culprits. Have some chicken, beef, lamb, liver, cheese, cauliflower, or broccoli.

- Salty Foods: Your body is craving silicon. So, go grab a few nuts and seeds; just be sure to count them into your daily counts.

Step 7: Learn the Basics of Meal Prep – Batching

You can not only save a lot of time, but you will also save a lot of money and carbs! So, let's get to it.

You're going to need plastic wrap, tin foil, wax paper, and lots of food storage containers. The best ones are clear, so when they're stacked in the fridge; you can tell what the contents are without any guesswork. Mason jars are also an excellent choice and a lot of fun for salads; you can layer different colored vegetables in them and then just add dressing and shake, it doesn't get much easier than that, plus, it's just so darn fancy.

Roasted Vegetables: By roasting veggies, you are not only able to quickly prepare them bulk, but you can also roast them on the same pan with a layer of tin foil. It is a good idea to prep 3 or 4 different veggies for one week, so you have a variety to go along with your new keto diet plan.

Barbecued Dishes: Anytime you barbecue food, it is going to be excellent for prepping. This is especially true of chicken, and no one ever minds eating it more than once each week. A pan of roasted chicken breasts can be spiced up using lemon pepper and BBQ seasoning. Just divide the two halves in the pan with a sheet of tin foil, and you've just cut away 45 min. off your cooking time.

About Seasoning. This will be your savior; it's a quick and easy way to jazz up any meal. You can add it to meats, vegetables, and carbs. It requires minimal effort and can take a 'blah' meal to a 'yum' meal in seconds. Garlic, lemon, rosemary, thyme, and sage; all pack a flavor punch, so go ahead and experiment with some different choices.

Always Make Protein Your Base for Prep. If there was a sale on chicken or fish, prepare 3 different flavors of that protein. You don't have to cook tuna, salmon, chicken, and turkey all at once, that's just exhausting, it's much easier to make 1 protein and just change up the spices so that it seems like you're getting three different items.

Bulk Prep the Carbs. Make a large pot of lentils, beans or quinoa; then you can either divide it into 2 or 3 different flavors with your herbs and spices or space it out over your containers and add a sauce to finish it off.

Now, another note of caution.

Don't Over-Prep. While you certainly don't want to run out of meals or short yourself on portions; you don't want to make so much food that you end up throwing it away. Not only is it wastefully expensive, but it's also eating into your free time since you had to cook all of the extras. Look at a reasonable portion size for you. If you know you'll eat 1 chicken breast per meal, then prep enough chicken breast for each meal you intend to have it for. Make 10, not 15.

Think about variety and options, such as boiled eggs; they are quick, easy and versatile. Add in precut raw veggies for snacking, mixing it up by including proportioned servings of cottage cheese or cut pieces of fruit, like apples along with the small premeasured packets of peanut or almond butter. These all make great go-to snacks either for between meetings at work, for the kids on the way to soccer practice or if you're just feeling a 'wee bit' of hunger between meals.

Step 8: Refine Your Meal Preparation Techniques

If you are hurrying all week long, it is a pleasant thought when you know you can go home and have your basic needs covered for dinner. You now understand how using basic meal prep - combined your new recipes help you remain in ketosis. Try the following methods.

Eggs

You can hard-boil the eggs to last for a week and store them in the refrigerator. The simplest way to know when you made them is to store them in the original container. Leave the shells on and mark the carton with the date and time. You can also use them in sandwiches or with a salad – anytime!

The reason to refrain from peeling the eggs is that they can absorb and create smells and mix flavors in the fridge. You don't want that to happen - so be sure the container used is airtight. Just place the whole carton into a zip-lock type bag for safe and easy access.

Meal Prep Ground Meats

Prepare the ground up meat by heating up a pan. Break the meat apart and cook until it's thoroughly done and browned. Give it 2-3 minutes to cool down. Prepare the packages into 3-ounce serving portions. Add them to airtight containers.

The prepared beef will not have a shelf-life of more than 3 days in the refrigerator. Before then, add the portions into freezer bags, making sure to remove as much air out the bag as you can before sealing. Enjoy the packaged meats for tacos, bun-less burgers, casseroles, or any other time you enjoy red meats.

It is vital to remove the ground meat from the store packaging quickly. Raw burger doesn't last as long as cooked portions. When it's time to thaw any frozen pieces, for safety reasons, thaw in the refrigerator, not the microwave. By doing it this way, the meat will last at least another day during the process. Doing so will keep the meat safe to use for an additional day or two.

Meal Prep Chicken

Before you get started, set the oven temperature to 350°F. Prepare a seasoning mixture of your choice. Cover the chicken with 1-2 tablespoons of oil and apply the seasonings. Place in the heated oven and cook approximately 30 minutes.
For a change of pace, use different types of seasonings on about half of the chicken. Use a sheet of aluminum foil to separate the flavors, so they don't combine. After the chicken has been cooked, be sure to let it cool down. Prepare it with a sharp knife into 3-ounce cuts and place the meat in multiple containers
awaiting a favorite veggie or dessert if you are doing complete meal prep.
Keep in mind; cooked chicken cannot last a week in the refrigerator. After 2-3 days, just dice or slice up any of the prepared meat. Add them into portions that
you believe you will use (3-oz. is a good guideline.). Arrange them in a high-quality freezer bag. Remove all air and close securely. Freeze until needed.

If you purchase breasts of chicken because they are the leanest cuts, you might want to reconsider for the meal prep process. Consider using chicken thighs, especially if you are on a budget. The fat content is slightly higher, but that is an advantage because they won't as easily dry out in the fridge.

It is vital to understand that it is not safe to reheat chicken more than once. Only warm up portions you can eat in one sitting. Chicken is best reheated the way it was cooked. Spread out the thawed chicken on a baking tin. Warm up the oven until it reaches 450°F. Cover with aluminum foil and bake for about 10 minutes.

Fruit Prep

<u>Apples</u>

You can enjoy apples at any time. They are low-maintenance for snacks or in a salad. Keep a stash of stashed in a crisper drawer for up to 4 weeks. All you need to do is slice, dice, or chop to your liking. You can prevent oxidization and browning by placing them in a glass dish filled with cold water.

Give the apples an extra boost by placing them on a damp paper towel in the refrigerator. The additional moisture helps them stay fresh longer. You can also put them in sealed plastic bags to keep them from being exposed to other fruits or vegetables that might have seepage of ethylene gas when released, resulting in spoilage.

<u>Bananas</u>

Use a few simple techniques to keep your bananas fresh longer. Begin the process as soon as you arrive home from the market. Take all them out of the plastic bags and separate each of the bananas from the bunch. Wrap them each stem of the bananas in a piece of plastic wrap and place it in the refrigerator. The wrap will hinder the ripening process from browning too quickly. The coldness will help keep the fruit firm.

You can also peel and slice them into 1-inch chunks. Add them to a sheet of parchment paper and place in the freezer. After they are frozen, store them in freezer bags. You can use these in smoothies, ice cream or baked goods, smoothies.

<u>Berries</u>

Are you surprised to see berries on a meal prep list? Many berries are notorious for spoiling easily. Don't worry there's an easy way to keep them fresh all week. Add three cups of water to one cup of vinegar in a large mixing container, Soak the berries in the mixture for about five minutes. Drain and pat them until they're as dry as you can get them. Store them in an airtight container lined with paper towels. Leave a crack the lid open to keep letting moisture escape.

Choose blueberries and strawberries over blackberries or raspberries. To prevent bruising, attempt to keep them in a single layer rather than piling them on top of each other.

<u>Grapes</u>

If stored correctly, grapes can last up to two to three weeks. Prepare an open container with a paper towel and arrange the grapes on top. The sheet will help draw out any extra moisture from the fruit and keep out bacteria and mold growth. Store the grapes in the coldest part of your fridge.

For the longest-lasting results, don't rinse the grapes until you're ready to eat them. Even if you do, you can still keep for up to a week if refrigerated.

Dessert is usually everyone's favorite part of the day. Why deny yourself? When you proportion out your servings, there are no fears that you'll demolish an entire the entire double chocolate cake. While 100 calorie packs are great but why get a little adventurous, you're already in the kitchen, how about a quick blender fruit puree, portioned out into a Tupperware container, for a refreshing treat later; or peanut/almond butter and thinly sliced fruit on graham crackers, you can slide them in a baggie and keep them in the fridge, perfect for a late night snack or if you're in an on the go rush; you can even get a little wild and sprinkle the peanut/almond butter with mini dark chocolate chips.

Step 9: Use intermittent fasting methods while using your ketogenic techniques.

Your metabolic rate is increased with short-term fasting because of the hormonal changes ranging in categories of 3.6% to 14%. Studies have established weight loss after three to twenty-four weeks on the intermittent fasting program to maintain losses of 3.0 to 8.0%. In comparison to other studies on weight loss, these are high percentages that cannot be ignored.

In the same studies, many of the individuals lost 4.0 to 7.0% of his/her waist circumference. This is an indication of how the harmful buildup of belly fat can cause disease and other issues around your organs. You have to consider these results are from eating fewer overall calories, and not binging during the days off. You have to maintain a sensible eating program.

While the core ideas behind the various forms of intermittent fasting are all the same, there are quite a few different ways to go about it. Your best bet is to try a few and see which one your body naturally responds to the easiest.

16:8 Method

This method involves fasting for 16 hours for men, or 14 hours for women, before allowing a reasonable number of calories for the remaining 8 to 10 hours. During this period, you should only consume items that have zero calories including black coffee (a splash of cream is okay), water, diet soda, and sugar-free gum. The easiest way to attempt this schedule is to stop eating after dinner in the evening and wait 14 or 16 hours from there. This means skipping breakfast and picking things up in the early afternoon.

Again, the specifics of when you fast are not nearly as important as ensuring that you fast for the same period of time as regularly as possible. If you vary your fasting period too much, it can lead to an erratic change in your hormones, which among other things; make it much more difficult for your body to shed any excess weight. If you find yourself without the time required to eat a proper meal to break the fast with a regular meal - you must eat something to keep your body on the correct cycle.

If you are exercising, as well as intermittently fasting, it is critical to ensure that you are eating more carbohydrates than fats while you are working out, while on days you are not exercising the opposite is true. It is vital to ensure - every day you keep your protein intake at a steady level. Stay away from processed foods whenever possible.

One of the most significant benefits of this type of fasting is that it's incredibly flexible so that it will work for a variety of schedules. Most people find it helpful to either eat two large meals during the 8 or 10-hour period feeding period or split that time into three smaller meals as that is the way most people are already programmed.

On days you are exercising as well as fasting, it is essential to try and always break your fast with a mix of protein, vegetables, and fruit. If you generally go to the gym directly after you have broken your fast, it is important to include enough carbohydrates to give your muscles the energy they need to get the most out of your workout.

If you are planning to exercise, it is usually best to start the early afternoon healthy with a medium calorie meal. Then, just exercise within three hours prior to consuming a more substantial meal soon afterward. In this meal, it is essential to add a substantial portion of complex carbohydrates. You can even have a little dessert as long as it is in moderation. Remember, fasting is different than dieting.

On days you do not plan on exercising, it is important to adjust your caloric intake appropriately. Start by limiting your carbohydrate intake, and instead focus on eating lots of protein, dark green, leafy vegetables and fruit in moderation. Unlike on days you are exercising, the first meal you eat on rest days should be your largest regarding caloric intake with this one meal counting for about 40 percent of your daily total.

Remember, during this meal, you should be taking in more protein than anything else. For your final meal during the 'rest' days; it's essential to include a protein source that will take lots of time to digest which in turn means it will keep you full for more of your fast the following morning. It also provides the body with enough stored amino acids to prevent it from breaking down muscle during the fast.

Eat-Stop-Eat

This form of fasting can be considered the most beneficial to those who are already eating healthy but want to give their weight loss an extra boost. On this type of program, you don't eat anything one or two days a week. During this period, you should only consume things that have zero calories including black coffee (a splash of cream is fine), water, diet soda, and sugar-free gum.

When you are finished fasting, it is important not to overeat more than average and always to avoid binging for extended periods of fast/binge cycles can cause severe damage to your body. As always, it is important to practice moderation and self-control to get the most out of the fasting cycle.

This fast cycle works on the assumption that in to lose a pound of weight a week, all you need to do is give up 3,500 calories. So, it might be best to get it out of the way in two quick bursts rather than fasting for a portion of every single day. This fasting plan emphasizes resistance weight training for maximum benefits.

Going a full day without eating can be difficult for some people at first, but it is perfectly acceptable to work up to a full day of fasting by holding out as long as possible and increasing that amount of time with practice. An excellent way to start is by choosing days that you know don't have any prior food commitments. Beginning a fasting program on a day when you know you have a lunch meeting is just a bad idea.

When first starting this fast cycle, fatigue, headaches or feelings of anger or anxiousness are all common side-effects and should be considered a good stopping point for your current fast. These side-effects will diminish as your body adjusts to the new cycle.

After going a full day without any calories, it will be natural to have the desire to binge during your first meal. You must have the self-control to fight these urges since not only is binging bad for you; it can quickly undo all of your hard work from the previous 24 hours. Practice self-discipline and make your fasting worth the effort.

The Warrior Diet

The Warrior Diet takes the 16:8 Program and kicks it up a notch by recommending that you fast for roughly 20 hours out of each day followed by one meal where you get all of your calories in the four remaining hours of the day.

This form of intermittent fasting follows the belief that humans are naturally nocturnal eaters. Therefore, eating at night helps the body more efficiently process the nutrients it needs. In this case, fasting is a bit of a misnomer as during the 20-hour period you are allowed to eat a serving of raw vegetables or fruits and maybe a serving of protein if you just can't otherwise continue.

This works because it causes the body's natural sympathetic nervous system to activate a flight or fight response which in turns increases your natural levels of alertness and increases energy while at the same time increasing the amount of fat burned. The large meal each evening then allows the body to focus on repairing itself and improving its muscles. When following the Warrior Diet, it is important to start each evening meal with vegetables, followed by protein, fat, and carbohydrates.

This form of fasting is famous for two reasons. First, the fact that a few small and reasonable snacks are allowed during the fasting process making this type of fasting attractive to those who are attempting the practice for the first time. Second, nearly everyone who tries this form of fasting reports a significant amount of increased energy throughout the day as well as an increase in the amount of fat lost per week.

On the other hand, the relatively strict nature of this diet can make it difficult for some people to follow for long periods of time. The timing of the large meal can also make it difficult for some people to follow because it can naturally interfere with some social engagements. Finally, some people don't like having to eat their food in a specific order. Try it for yourself and see what works for you.

Fat Loss Forever

This form of intermittent fasting combines elements of several other styles of fasting to create something somewhat unique. The good news is that you get a cheat day every week. The bad news is that it is followed by a one and a half day fast with the remainder of the week being split between 16:8 and 20:4 fasting.

For this diet, it is important to schedule your exercise rest days for the second part of the 36-hour cycle. Otherwise, it is essential to stay as busy on these days as possible to help combat your hunger. If you find it hard to control your appetite on cheat days, then this form of intermittent fasting may not be for you since it requires you to go from sixty to zero quickly and regularly.

Also, it is important not to try and last 36 hours without eating food all at once. You will need to build up your body's tolerance for fasting. As such, it is usually better to start with another form of intermittent fasting and work up to the Fat Loss Forever method after your body has already gotten out of the habit of eating every three or four hours.

Remember always to fast responsibly, and never push your body to the point where you feel physically ill. Also, remember it is essential to fast on a routine to allow your body the time it needs to adjust to the change.

Alternate Day Diet

This form of intermittent fasting actually means you never have to go long without food, if you so choose. Every other day you eat as usual, and on the off-days, you merely consume one-fifth of the calories you take in on the regular days. The average daily caloric consumption is between 2,000 and 2,500 calories which mean that the regular off-day varies between 400 and 500 calories. If you enjoy exercising every day, then this form of intermittent fasting may not be for you since you will have to limit your workouts on off-days severely.

When you first start this form of intermittent fasting, the easiest way to make it through the low-calorie days is by trying any one of a variety of protein shakes. It is important to work back to 'real' natural foods on these days because they will always be healthier than the shakes.

This form of intermittent fasting is all about losing weight. Those who try it tend to average between two and three pounds lost per week. If you attempt the Alternate Day Diet, it is imperative to eat regularly on your full-calorie days. Binging will not only negate any progress you have made, but it can also cause severe damage to your body if continued over time.

Irregularly Skipping Meals

If you are interested in trying out the benefits of intermittent fasting for yourself, but you have an irregular schedule or are not sure if it is for you, then skipping a meal or two now and then maybe the type of intermittent fasting for you. As previously discussed, getting into a fasting routine is vital to see the maximum results for your effort, but that doesn't occasionally mean fasting doesn't come with some benefits as well.

What's more, once you have tried skipping a meal now and then you can see for yourself just how easy it is which in turn can lead to more positive changes down the line. With so many intermittent fasting options available the odds are good that one fits your schedule, so give it a try. What have you got to lose (besides a few pounds)?

Chapter 7: How to Know If You Are in Ketosis

Maintaining ketosis is an individual process, and you need to be sure you are achieving your goals. The levels of acetone, acetoacetate, and beta-hydroxybutyrate can be measured in your breath, urine, and blood.

You can measure the ketones with a blood ketone meter which works similar to a glucose meter. Add a small drop of blood on a testing strip and insert the tab into the meter. It will indicate the amount of beta-hydroxybutyrate in your bloodstream. This process has been researched as a valid indicator of the current ketosis levels. Unfortunately, the strips are expensive.

Test your urine for acetoacetates. The strip is dipped into the urine which will change the color of the testing strip. The various shades of purple and pink indicate the levels of the ketones. The darker the color on the testing strip; the higher the level of ketones in your body. The primary benefit is; they are inexpensive. The most effective time to test is during the early morning hours - after a ketogenic diet dinner the evening before testing.

You should use one or more of these methods to indicate whether you need to adjust your intake of foods to remain in ketosis.

Option 1: The Ketone Testing Process with Your Breath

One of the ketones that will present itself to be measured is produced by gas exchanging in your lungs to create acetate or acetone. This causes you to breathe out a measurable level of ketones.

The levels can be measured directly through the breath with the use of a Ketonix device to measure the breath acetone or

BrAce which measures in parts per million (ppm). There are a few different Ketonix devices that are preprogrammed to show different colors of lights blinking at different frequencies depending what levels of BrAce ppm are in your blood and have companion apps that run on your computer. The ketonix meter is reusable and just a one-time purchase unlike urine or blood strips, which are one-time use.

Once you purchase your ketonix meter; the only requirement is to plug it into the included battery pack or into a USB port. It may take a few minutes to activate, but all you need to do is blow into the unit until it begins flashing to read the levels of acetone in your breath. The codes are as follows:
- Green color: Least amounts of acetone
- Red color: More volumes of accumulated acetone

The number of times the color tone is flashing:
- Less color flashing: Means less acetone per color level
- More color flashing: Means more acetone per color

Note: The number and color codes used with the flashing options will provide accurate measurements of the levels of acetone levels. If you use them, it's best to correlate with blood meter until you have discovered your baselines.

Advantages of testing ketosis levels with a breath meter:
- Reusable device.
- Doesn't use bodily fluids

Disadvantages of using a breath meter for testing ketosis levels with a breath meter:
- Inaccurate measurement of acetone levels
- Indirect measurement of the current levels of acetone
- Inconsistent reading of the acetone levels
- Takes a much longer than urine or blood tests to get a reading

Option 2: The Ketone Testing Process with Urine Strips:

The way to measure these excess amounts of ketones is through a simple urine strip. The strip changes colors relative to the number of ketones in your urine, and you can have a general idea of what level the ketones are in excess.

One of the enormous advantages of testing ketone levels using a urine strip is that is very easy and very cheap to do. The price is usually under $10 for a package of 100 testing strips.

Taking the test is pretty straightforward. You can do it anytime and anywhere you think you might have steered out of ketosis.

Option 3: The Ketone Testing Process with A Blood Meter

Testing levels of ketones by looking at amounts of beta-hydroxybutyrate may be accomplished by sampling the blood. This can be done quickly at home the same way individuals with diabetes check their blood glucose. Prick your finger, squeeze a drop of blood and press it on the testing strip. The machine will let you know if you are still in line with your levels of ketosis.

Unlike the urine test, your blood is a very tightly regulated system and doesn't get diluted or change with different factors of hydration making this is the most direct way to measure the level of ketosis.

The disadvantage is many individuals have a dislike of needles. If you are on a budget, you also have to consider the strips are significantly expensive, usually $5-$10 per testing strip which can add up quickly.

Chapter 8: Diet & Exercise: The Right Combination

Combining the diet with exercise is the combination you can have for best weight loss results. Activity is an essential component to the success or failure of the ketogenic diet plan. You produce cortisol which is a hormone released from your adrenal gland in response to chemical signs or other stress signals. The release of cortisol in long workouts and jogging are essential elements in your weight loss program.

Maintaining ketosis can be easily accomplished once you have your plan in gear. You need to exercise and watch your diet. It takes time to get it right, so don't get discouraged. This segment will provide you some insight on how to get going and keep it going.

Provide the Balance

Short exercises of approximately 21 minutes daily have been scientifically proven more beneficial than longer workouts. By combining the right diet with the proper training, you can get into shape without a lot of fancy equipment.

When you are pumping away on a stationary bike or treadmill, you're building up the cortisol in your body. Cortisol is a stress hormone that usually helps burn fat. However, if you have stressful and lengthy exercises planned, your body will move into a protection mode which will cause storage of fat around your midsection. That can put you at risk for cancer, diabetes, or heart disease.

For success. It is best to use a high-intensity interval training (HIIT) method. You can work-out in short intervals during a lunch break or any part of the day you feel the need to get moving.

A Beginner Regimen for Your Exercise Plan

Monday:

Begin your week out using 30-minute workouts for your lower body weight.
Perform 5 sets of 5 repetitions of:
- Squats
- Deadlifts
- Lunges

Finish off the time with a walk on the treadmill.

Tuesday:

After your stressful workout on Monday, just take today off and do a little break time with some yoga or other relaxation methods. Clear your head and enjoy one of your delicious snack time treats.

Wednesday:

It is back to work time with a 30-minute upper body weight training session. Workout using five sets of five repetitions of each:
- Shoulder press
- Dumbbell rows
- Bench press

Thursday:

Have a low-intensity day. Try going for a 30 to 45-minute walk somewhere that is quiet and peaceful. Keep your stress levels at a minimum.

Friday:

Have a day of rest. Consider planning one of your weekly ketogenic meals, so you are ahead of the game. Think of all of the delicious treats that await you.

Saturday:

Go for a strenuous - 45-minute to one-hour training regimen using your full body weight training techniques. Workout using five sets and five repetitions of these:
- Squats
- Bench Press or Pushups with more reps.
- Barbell rows
- Lunges

Sunday:

As many have practiced for years, take a day of rest any way you choose. Relax is the key!

You have some suggestions of how to burn away those pounds. These are several ways to jazz it up!

Have Some Fun: Go Swimming:

Swimming is a favorite cardio workout because your entire body is burning calories. This is a fantastic plus since it works your whole body, burning away calories. Swimming allows you to 'work' all of your significant muscles without taxing unnecessary impact on your joints. It is just as popular as walking for many individuals.

Try Power Walking:

An hour of daily brisk walking is fantastic for boosting your metabolism and stress reduction. It is excellent for loosening up the hips and hamstrings, relaxing any tension and reversing the detrimental effects of sitting at a desk all day.

Super Tips for Keto and Your Exercise Routine

Go Slow at First.

The professionals suggest you don't attempt to change too many things too quickly. If you have been inactive or eating as many individuals do in today's society, it may take some time to get your body adjusted. Go slowly.

You might not feel exhilarated at first. Try not to let this have an effect on your workouts. You may also feel like you're in a fog for a day or so when you combine your ketogenic diet with your workout methods. Luckily, the mental dullness will typically pass after a few days, but the professionals suggest to limit workouts that require quick reactions to remain safe, such as going for a ride on your bicycle on heavily traveled roads with cars.

Always Listen to Your Body

During the first few weeks on your new way of eating, your body is making a lot of changes. If you feel overwhelmed, maybe it is time to reconsider whether the dieting method you are using is working as it should. Try adjusting the number of carbs you eat daily. Eat a bit more often. If these suggestions don't work, maybe it is time to speak with your doctor.

Add Some Natural Supplements to Your Plan

Bone Broth: This treat has been around for many years. The broth can eliminate keto flu symptoms and provide you with an increase of your essential electrolytes. These are just several of the benefits:

- Boosting your immune system
- Keeping your intestinal tract healthier

- Increases collagen levels to improve your eyes, heart, skin, joints, and bone. You will also achieve improved brain health.

Make you a batch anytime to sip or use in your cooking. Use the recipe below:

Yields: 6-8 cups
Prep & Cooking Time: 6 hours – 45 minutes
Nutrients Per Cup: 0.7 g Net Carbs | 72 Cal. | 3.6 g Protein| 6 g Fat

Ingredients:
- 3 ½ lb. mixed assorted bones – ex. marrow bones, chicken feet or your choice
- 1 tbsp. pink Himalayan salt
- 1 med. of each:
  -Parsnip
  -White onion – skin on
- 5 peeled garlic cloves
- 2 med. of each:
  -Celery stalks
  -Carrots
- 2 tbsp. lemon juice or apple cider vinegar
- 8 c. of water
- Slow Cooker

Method:
1. Peel and slice the vegetables with roots into 1/3-inch pieces. Slice the onion in half. Chop the celery into thirds. Add the bay leaves into the slow cooker.
2. Toss in the chosen bones (can also be pork). Pour the water up to ¾ capacity – along with the juice/vinegar, and bay leaves. Sprinkle with the salt.
3. Secure the lid. Choose either low (ten hours) or high (six hours). You can simmer up to 48 hours.
4. Use a strainer to remove the bits of veggies. Set the

bones aside to chill. Shred the meat and use as desired.

5. Refrigerate the broth overnight. Scrape away the fat layer if desired. Use within five days or freeze. You can also keep it in the canning jars for up to 45 days.

Fermented Foods: Foods such as coconut water kefir or coconut milk kefir, pickles, sauerkraut, and kimchi are beneficial to your digestive system. The natural acids also help stabilize your blood sugar levels as well as the enzymes, probiotics, and other bioactive nutrients help support ketosis. These are three excellent reasons you should consume fermented foods.
Fermented foods help restore the 'good' bacteria in your guy.

Probiotics: You can eat kimchee, Greek yogurt, kefir or similar fermented foods. You can also take a supplement.

Apple Cider Vinegar (ACV): A typical carbohydrate meal can be reduced by 31% with the use of this acetic acid by reducing the glycemic response. ACV also contains enzymes that will enhance the metabolism of fats and proteins.

You can add it full-strength or use an 8-ounce glass of water with 1 to 2 tablespoons of vinegar. These are some of the ways you can benefit from consuming ACV:

- Improves digestion
- Strengthens your immune system
- Great for detoxification
- Reduces cholesterol
- Good energy booster
- Helps you lose weight
- Helps relieve sore muscles
- Aids in diabetes/controls blood sugar
- Balances your inner body system

Lemon and Lime: These are two citric acid filled supplements to consider to reduce your blood sugar levels naturally. The trace minerals in lemon and lime, such as potassium, are present to improve your insulin—signaling a boost in your liver function.

You can use them in many ways including overcooked veggies or meats, in your green juices, or with your salad to improve your state of ketosis.

- Boosts your immune system
- Blood purifier
- Balances pH
- Reduces fever
- Flushes out unwanted materials
- Excellent for weight loss
- Decreases blemishes and wrinkles
- Relieves respiratory infections
- Reduces toothache pain

Turmeric: The use or this Asian orange herb dates back to Ayurveda and Chinese medicine. The curcumin (an anti-inflammatory compound) found in the turmeric helps improve your insulin receptor function while regulating your blood sugar levels. Add turmeric to your meats, vegetables, green drinks, or smoothies. To maximize the antioxidant elements, add the turmeric after the meal is finished cooking.

Turmeric has many health benefits:

- Weight Management
- Prevents Alzheimer's Disease
- Relieves Arthritis
- Controls Diabetes
- Reduces the Cholesterol Level
- Improves digestion

Other Supplements for Ketosis

The ketogenic diet has many benefits, but it's possible some of the essential nutrients are being overlooked in your menu planning. You may need to supplement to replace minerals including magnesium, potassium, calcium, and sodium which comes from some of the food items not used on the keto diet. These electrolytes control muscle and nerve function and many other issues. Below are just a few of the ways you can supplement your plan:

The Electrolytes: If you have a low level of electrolytes, especially potassium and sodium, you can frequently suffer from fatigue, headaches, and constipation which is commonly called keto flu. The low-carbs also cause the kidneys to dump excess water, sodium and other valuable electrolytes that much be replenished.

Magnesium: One of the most evident signs of a deficiency in magnesium is muscle cramps and fatigue. A blood test is the best way to test for possible problems. Magnesium has many benefits including proper nerve and muscle function, helps maintain normal heart rhythm, assists over 300 body reactions including supporting adequate testosterone levels and working with calcium to keep your bones healthy.

Ideally, men should consume 420 mg. daily; women need only 320 mg. Eat some of these foods to maintain adequate magnesium levels:
* Leafy green vegetables
* Pumpkin seeds
* Avocados
* Almonds
* High-fat yogurts

Sodium: The amount of sodium required differs from other diet plans because other plans generally focus on less sodium. The sodium is lost with the water loss so you will need to increase the sodium intake to keep the right balance of electrolytes. This is crucial especially during the initial phase of the diet. Gain sodium in these ways:

- Drinking bone broth regularly
- Adding salt to your food - Himalayan sea salt is a good choice.
- Enjoy more sodium-rich foods including eggs and red meats
- Be sure to monitor your blood pressure because the sodium can have an effect on your pressure levels if you're are prone to hypertension.

Potassium: Your normal blood pressure, regular heart rate, and fluid balance are aided by potassium. You need to remain cautious about adding potassium supplements to your diet because too much can cause an overload which could be toxic. Eat the following foods instead:

- Salmon
- Mushrooms
- Avocados
- Leafy greens
- Nuts

Calcium: Strong bones, muscle contraction, and proper blood clotting are all elements involved with calcium. Use these sources to add to your calcium counts:

- Leafy greens such as broccoli
- Dairy & non-dairy milk – unsweetened & zero carbs

You may need to supplement with calcium supplements including Vitamin D which is necessary for absorption. Both women and men should consume approximately 1000 mg. daily of calcium.

Vitamin D: Nutrients and hormones in your body are supplied by Vitamin D. You cannot always get enough from your food, but you can go outside and take in some fresh sunshine for your portion. Use caution from over-exposure and the risks of skin cancer. The D vitamin also helps your body to absorb magnesium, calcium and other essential minerals to maintain your muscle growth and bone density. If yours' is low; you are like about 1/3 of all Americans.

Supplement by adding 400 IU per day as recommended and add some fatty fish and mushrooms to your diet plan.

Fish Oil: Purchase this at any health food store in either the liquid or capsule form. The oil provides a natural anti-inflammatory content and also contributes to the higher fat intake requirements on the ketogenic diet.

MCT Oils: Your ketogenic experience can improve with the use of MCT oil or medium chain triglycerides. These fatty acids are found in its natural form in palm and coconut oil. Its advantages include:

- The oil helps lower your blood sugar.
- The use of MCTs makes it much easier to get into – and remain in ketosis. It is a natural anti-convulsive.
- It is also excellent for appetite control and weight loss.

Chlorella: The green algae superfood is good for fighting off fatigue. It contains Chlorella Growth Factor – a nutrient containing DNA and RNA to help increase energy transport between your cells. You can purchase the supplement in powder form, tablets, or capsules. Mix it with water, one of your new smoothies, or other drinks. Have one daily.

Spirulina: The blue-green algae is similar to chlorella and contains all the amino acids your body requires which makes it a complete protein. It also contains magnesium, iron, potassium and other beneficial nutrients. It has superb antioxidant properties. The medication has shown positive results with individuals who suffer from cholesterol and high blood pressure. It will raise the good cholesterol or HDL and reduce the bad cholesterol or LDL. You can purchase it in capsule form or in powder to mix in water or with a tasty smoothie.

Acetyl L-Carnitine: The carnitine helps your muscle cells to force or drive energy proficiently from fat metabolism because a lower level of the carnitine causes a reduced ability to use fat for energy. You need to keep the levels up to remain in ketosis.

CoQ10: Coenzyme Q10 is the technical term for this powerful antioxidant. It is also a central molecule in your cellular process of creating energy. You can supplement your diet with 100 to 300 mg each day.

Creatine: This amino acid is favored by bodybuilders and athletes. It can be purchased either from a health food store or online with Amazon. Its most beneficial feature is for strengthening and building lean muscle mass as well as enhancing athletic performance.

Glutamine: Eight grams daily—taken orally—immediately after your workout—can help promote the production of glucose during exercise. When you purchase glutamine, don't buy the powders because they usually have additives or sugar content.

Greens/Veggie Supplements: The best way to get the greens in your keto diet is through meals such as spinach in your eggs or a low-carb veggie juice with a cheese snack. Have a salad with dinner. However, if you don't like greens; you can purchase a greens supplement. A measured scoop of a protein shake will help with the issue.

Perfect Keto: You can use this powdered drink supplement to help spike your ketone levels. Don't be mistaken; this cannot replace the keto diet plan. It is a good stand-by if you exceed your carb limit. It can only assist to keep you in ketosis.

Vanadium and Chromium: Chromium and Vanadium are both trace minerals which are essential to the production of insulin which will stabilize your body's blood sugar level.

The Stalling and Plateaus of Weight Loss

At first, you may not notice the weight loss. There could be days or weeks where you don't see the changes, but slow is the best method. You are altering your lifestyle and breaking old habits. You need to remain patient because there aren't any quick fixes to weight loss.

As with any new challenge, the initial phase of a long-term challenge is difficult. Once you have discovered how easy the ketogenic plan is; you will wonder how it took you so long to try it.

Check Your Medications

It's important to inform your doctor of your weight loss program. He/she may prescribe some medicines that make you gain weight. These are a few to question:

Insulin Injections: If taken in high doses, your insulin can impede weight loss. By consuming fewer carbs, you are substantially reducing the requirement of insulin. Again, ask your healthcare professional before you make any changes.

Other Possible Medications Causing Weight Gain:

- Oral contraceptives
- Anti-Depressants
- Epilepsy drugs
- Blood pressure medications
- Allergy medicines
- Antibiotics

More Sleep & Less Stress

If you are a victim of sleep deprivation, you will understand how stressful everyday life is, even before you begin a diet plan. You may believe it's too late for you, but it isn't. Your diet plan will work, but you may need to make a few other adjustments.

Chronic stress will increase your cortisol levels – the stress hormone. With that action, your hunger levels also rise. The result is that you eat more and put on the weight. It's important to find ways to remove the stress; whether it is decluttering your home or taking a vacation.

Eliminate coffee or other forms of caffeine early in the afternoon and don't consume alcohol for at least three hours before bedtime. Alcohol can also interfere with your quality of sleep which is why you wake up feeling tired after an evening of nightclubs or boozing.

If you enjoy working out for your health, be sure to do that at least four hours before time for sleeping. Make sure your room is sufficient darkness. You will wake refreshed, ready to face your tasty ketogenic breakfast.

Weigh the Now and Later

It is always tempting to test your loyalty to the diet and exercise plan you have chosen. You will need to learn how to pass by that sweet treat you are craving. You'll be happier in the long-term by continuing on the right path to weight loss and not cheating with the loaded calories.

Chapter 9: Ketogenic Diet FAQs

Commonly Used Abbreviations

You may become overwhelmed as you browse the Internet for new ketogenic recipes. I have provided you with a few abbreviations you may not recognize.

These are a few:

- Bulletproof Coffee (*BPC*) is generally a mixture of coffee, oil, and butter. It is meant to give you a full feeling.
- Extra-virgin olive oil (EVOO)
- Heavy Whipping Cream (*HWC*) is used by many cooks.
- Low-carb and High-Fat (*LCHF*)
- Sugar-Free (*SF*)Artificial Sweetener (*AS)* provides a zero/reduced carb count.

You will be using EVOO for many of the recipes. You can make your own spray by adding the oil to a spray bottle. You can also use canola oil which is also an excellent choice for baking.

Frequently Asked Questions

Question #1: Who should avoid the Keto diet techniques? Before you make any decisions to begin the plan, consult your physician if you have suffered from any of the following:

- Impaired liver function
- History of pancreatitis
- Gallbladder related issues
- Gastric bypass surgery
- Impaired fat digestion
- History of kidney failure

- Women who are pregnant or lactating

At this point, you are making a meaningful change, and you should consult your personal dietitian or doctor for advice before moving forward.

Question #2: Do I need to know my 'ideal' body weight? The Body Measurements: Most people step on a scale every morning and hope to see a difference. Our bodies don't exactly work like that. Don't rely on numbers alone!

It is recommended that using a tape measure to track progress using the same points on your body week by week. For example, take the measurement of your waist once a week and track your progress in that way. The preferred method is just taking pictures. Over time, you'll see a huge difference. Focus on the long-term and remember, progress is slow and steady.

Tracking progress is critical because it acts as an anchor and shows you just how well you're doing. It'll motivate you to succeed too!

Question#3: How can I make the process easier? Prepare a Menu and Food Plan: Use some of the recipes in this book and combine them with your other ketogenic favorites. You will be surprised how many tasty items you can enjoy that are full of healthy nutrients.

Question #4: How can I remain optimistic? Begin Your New Lifestyle – Not Your New Diet: Most diets are not successful because they stay just that – diets. They are merely short-term solutions for long-term problems. Low carb is a lifestyle change which has been proven to be one of the healthiest ways to live. Make a commitment to this way of life and try to make your meals fast, simple and delicious. If you've got a game plan, you'll more likely stay on track.

Question #5: Do I need to stop eating regularly? "Don't Try to Starve Yourself." Another major misconception of dieting is that you have to starve yourself to see results and that can actually be damaging your long-term health. This is just not true with the methods used on the ketogenic plan.

Question #6: Is the Keto Diet a restrictive diet that tastes bad? Don't Restrict Your Diet Severely: Diet foods don't have to taste bad. This is one of the most common misconceptions about diets – people think that diet foods have to taste bad. It's just not right! Explore your options and discover all the delicious meals you can make a daily part of your life.

Chapter 10: Living the Keto Lifestyle

Only Eat When You're Hungry! One outstanding benefit of the keto diet plan is that you don't stay hungry which makes it a sustainable lifelong choice. This is a common mistake when people first start a new diet, but with the ketogenic method, you can have the fats. Carbs and fats are your two significant sources of energy for your body. If you are removing the carbs, they must be replaced by fats. Remove both elements, and you would starve. By consuming natural fats, you are satisfied. Enjoy eggs, fatty fish, coconut and olive oil, bacon, meat, butter, and full-fat cream.

When your body doesn't have insulin that stores the fat, you will become a fat-burning machine and start dropping those unwanted pounds. Trust your instincts and cut out one of the meals or eat several times a day - but keep track of the carbs.

Preparing Keto Meals on A Budget

I already mentioned meal prepping which is at the top of the list when you're on a budget. However, many more elements come into the game plan.

When you think of the ketogenic diet, typical foods that come to mind probably include chicken, steak, fatty fish such as salmon, and even bacon. Buying these foods can quickly get expensive. But, there are ways to do it without breaking the bank. The keto diet can definitely be done on a budget. When possible, it is always best to begin by purchasing quality over quantity.

If you're not mindful of quality and give in to eating processed cheese, low-quality meats, or foods full of additives and preservatives, it could counterbalance the ketones in your bloodstream and disrupt your diet.

Here are nine ways to save money while doing the ketogenic diet, from shopping locally to buying whole chickens rather than individual sections such as breasts and thighs.

1. Shop Locally. When possible purchase your produce and other items directly from the farmer, either by visiting local farmers' markets or farm.

2. Buy in Bulk. *Buying certain foods in bulk is a crucial way to keep costs down.*
Buying in bulk is key to doing the keto diet on a budget, especially when it comes to meat. You can always partner with other family or friends to do share purchasing a whole cow. Consider investing in an additional freezer in your garage.

You could also save money by getting your nuts, seeds, and coconut oil in bulk from health food stores online.

3. Purchase whole chickens instead of just chicken breasts. Buy whole chickens, slow cook or roast, and put left-overs in the fridge or freezer, since it's much cheaper than merely buying only the chicken breasts.

Don't worry about the process taking too much time out of your busy schedule. There is a simple trick you can use called spatchcocking. All you need to do is split the chicken by removing its backbone. The time is reduced to 30 minutes since the chicken is spread flay as it is being cooked. This is how it's done:

1. Arrange the chicken on a baking tin or cutting board with the breast side facing downward.
2. Use a sharp pair of kitchen scissors to cut away the backbone. Start at the thigh and work your way up the back.
3. Flip the chicken over (breast side upward) and press it flat.
4. That is all there is to it!

4. Stock up on eggs. Eggs are a valuable protein food and can be added to so many delicious recipes. Prepare hard-boiled for your morning meal or throw some into a salad as a great way to get your protein for less money.

5. Buy in-season vegetables. Buying vegetables that are in-season can save you money. When you purchase what is in season, you are buying food that's at the peak of its supply, and it costs less for farmers and distribution companies to harvest it and get it to the store.

6. Buy vegetables in bulk and freeze them. As an example, avocados can be expensive, but if you come across some that are discounted because they're about to be past their sell-by date, you can buy them and freeze the flesh to use in smoothies.

7. Keep it simple. At first, if you're a beginner using the ketogenic dieting technique, it's always a good idea to keep things simple. Just build your plate from a medium-sized piece of protein, add some produce either cooked in or drizzled with fat. All of the recipes in this book are good examples of how simple it is to enjoy a healthy meal any time of the day or night.

Measure Your Food with Accuracy

Purchase a Food Scale:

Keeping accurate records is essential to know how many carbs, fats, and proteins you are consuming. Guesswork can be costly such as a 6-ounce steak could very well be an 8-ounce piece of meat. You have to be precise to keep your body in the right mode. These are some of the options you should consider when you buy a new food scale:

- Removable Plate: For health reasons, a removable plate will allow you to keep the germs at 'bay' for easy cleaning.

- Automatic Shut-off: Search for a scale that doesn't have an auto shut-off button. Nothing is more frustrating than to be adding your meal totals, and it shuts off!

- Have a Conversion Button: Many of the websites and recipe apps use different units of measure. It is beneficial to have one that can convert the ounces to grams for easy measuring of your food items.

- Tare Function: A tare feature will allow you to set the scale back to zero when you place plates, bowls, or other items on the weighing scale.

Purchase Helpful Gadgets

In today's society, you have so many useful appliances to use in your kitchen, cooking healthier is much easier, accurate, and quicker. This segment will enlighten you to some of those tools:

- Veggie Spiralizer: You can prepare tasty vegetables quickly and easily without the extra fuss.

- Measuring Cups & Spoons: Purchase a quality set of cups and spoons to ensure you are using exact measurements. Many of the recipes do not include the Metric and American standard sizes. It is best to save the time and have the information right there on your tools.

Use the Slow Cooker

Think of how many times you have experienced 'spells' that you did not feel like spending hours over the stove preparing dinner. Can you relate? How about the times during the holidays when you are planning on a houseful of guests; yikes? Don't worry because you have your fabulous cooker and all of these new recipes to experiment with in your kitchen. These are a few ways to make the path a bit easier:

Save a lot of Effort and Time: All it takes is a few good recipes and a little bit of your valuable time. In most of the cases, these recipes are geared towards a fast lifestyle and will be ready with just a few simple steps. After some time and practice, you will have a list of your favorites.

Get Ahead of the Meal: Preparing food with your slow cooker can put you ahead of the game. You can prepare the cooker the night before if you have a busy day planned. All it takes is a few minutes of preparation. Just add all of the fixings (if they can combine overnight) into the pot, so when you get up the next morning; all you need to do is take it out of the fridge, and let it get to room temperature. Turn it on as you head out of the door and dinner will be ready when you get home.

Cut Back on Dining Out: Having an enjoyable meal at home is so much more personal for your family because you prepared it! Not only that, you will eliminate the temptation to order foods that might not be so healthy and will also be more expensive than dining at home.

Watching the Extra Liquids: There is no need to use additional ingredients, other than what is described in each of the recipes. Ideally, you should not fill the crock pot more than half to two-thirds full of the fixings. Too much liquid will cause leakage from the top and may result in a poor-quality meal.

Cook it Slow & Leave it Alone: A slow cooker is known for creating delicious dishes while bringing out all of the natural flavors. So, go on about your busy schedule and don't worry! There is no need to worry about checking on it (unless the recipe calls for it). Each time the lid is removed—valuable heat is escaping—resulting in a breakdown of the advised times. Just keep that thought in mind, even though it is tempting to open the pot and smell the aromas!

Trimming the Fat: One huge advantage to the use of this type of cooking is you can save quite a chunk of money purchasing cheaper cuts of meat. Also, capitalize on the flavorful meat in small quantities and by bulking up on veggies with smaller meat portions.

Dining Out Tips

When you make a choice to dine out; be smart and do some online research before you leave the house. Many of the restaurants now have an online presence to make dieting a less daunting adventure. Try to plan your meals ahead of time when possible. These are a few recommendations that might help:

- **Breakfast:** Sometimes, there is nothing better than eggs if you want to play it safe. You may be off on some of the counts but after you have used some of the recipes in this book; you will know how to gauge your eating habits for the most important meal of the day.

- **Lunch:** Fish and Chicken are usually good choices. Many of the restaurants now offer diet-friendly menus. Try something like chicken salad or a regular salad. You need to beware of the dressing used. Try some vinaigrette or plain vinegar.

- **Dinner:** Always choose a fresh green veggie with a lean cut of meat as your main course. Try something in the line of a hamburger minus the bun, or a tempting entrée of broccoli and steak. Yummy!

Dining Choices – Be Aware

Wheat products contain an enormous amount of carbs. This will eliminate a pita or a tortilla as well as a plate of French fries. You will also be disappointed that you cannot have a baked potato either. Ask for a substitute with another side dish. Most restaurants will be happy to accommodate your request, especially if he/she knows you are on a particular diet plan.

Common Mistakes Using the Keto Diet.

Here are a few unfortunate choices made by dieters as reasons that could cause your diet to fail. Making changes to your diet should fit into your lifestyle, so the task doesn't need to become a dreaded chore; that is if you plan the route to success ahead of meal times.

You learn from your mistakes, and these are some of the ones that can happen along the path:

Mistake #1: Dieting Solo: Dieting is a challenge, but many individuals have discovered dieting with another friend, or family members can make the task seem less stressful. Many of the temptations can be removed if everyone is on the same page. You can also join a support group online or better yet – start your own team. The primary element is to be around individuals who understand your struggle. Praise of losing the pounds and inches while staying healthy is what the Keto diet plan is all about!

Mistake #2: Dining by the Clock: Just because the clock says it is 12:00 noon or 6:00 dinnertime doesn't mean you must have a meal. If you have in the past, you understand the pitfall. One crucial step while you are dieting is that you should never eat unless you are hungry. Take the clues from your body, not the clock.

Mistake #3: Becoming Obsessed with the Weighing Scales: Weighing often can sometimes cause setbacks, because you don't believe you are progressing as fast as you want to at this point. You have to realize the numbers you are viewing on the scales are from work done previously; not today. Your weight will fluctuate daily according to your water weight, so it is not as dependable as waiting for a week or more before you weigh.

Mistake #4: Obsessing Over the Macros: The keto diet plan takes a lot of the stress out of the process of counting the macros. It is a simple process to track the numbers, but try not to become obsessed with them.

Mistake #5: Lack of Commitment: You have to be ready to change your lifestyle and become determined to eat for your health. You have to commit yourself 100% to the plan to reap the promising results. Only you know how many grams of food you have consumed in one day. Be honest when recording your intake amounts.

Mistake #6: Lack of Essential Nutrients: According to the experts, you need to be getting salt in your diet daily. You need to consume a minimum of two teaspoons each day, as well as Vitamin D and magnesium while on the keto plan. Many of the nutrients are supplied through your foods.

Mistake #7: Eating the Wrong Types of Fat: You need to steer clear of seed and vegetable oils (many stored in plastic containers). Instead, purchase saturated fats such as butter, animal fats, or coconut oil, and monounsaturated fat such as olive oil, and fish oil.

Mistake #8: Consuming Too Much Protein: Protein provides an essential macro essential to building your muscles, organs, and other soft tissues. Your efforts to reach ketosis will be sabotaged if you consume too much protein. If you eat more than you need, the surplus will be transformed into glucose.

Mistake # 9: Comparison to Others: The success of this diet plan depends on what you believe is right and correct, not what others think is right. Everyone gains and loses weight differently; it isn't a one-size-fits-all situation. Just because a friend lost 30 pounds in 30 days, and you didn't; doesn't make you a failure. It merely means you have to become more diligent and try again.

Chapter 11: Ketogenic Recipes

This entire segment is dedicated to your recipes for breakfast, lunch, dinner, snacks, and desserts.

11.1: Breakfast Recipes

Bacon – Spinach - Avocado & Egg

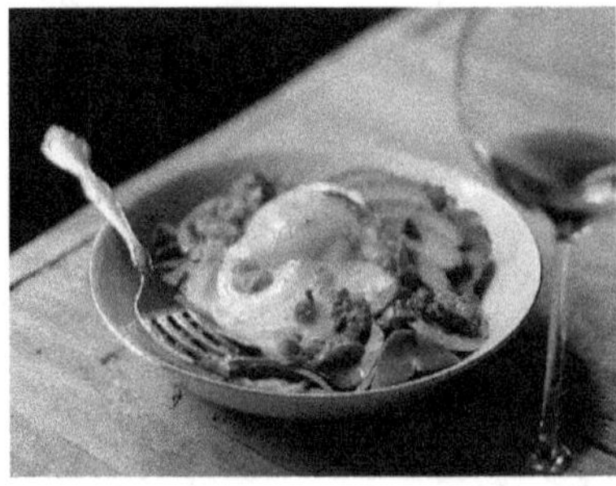

2 servings
Macronutrients: 33 g Protein | 57 g Fats |9 g Carbs|4 g Net Carbs

Ingredients:
- 2 large eggs
- 6 slices of bacon
- 2 tbsp. heavy whipping cream
- 1 tbsp. butter
- 1 cup fresh spinach or a favorite choice
- 1/2 sliced avocado
- To Taste:
  -Freshly cracked black pepper
  -Pink Himalayan salt

Method:

1. Use the medium heat setting on the stovetop to prepare the bacon – total of about 8 minutes.
2. Drain the grease on a towel-lined platter.
3. Whisk the cream, eggs, pepper, and salt. Add half to the skillet of grease. Cook until set (1 min.) and flip. Add more butter if needed. Prepare the second egg - cooking 1 more minute per side. Drain on a paper towel.
4. Serve on a warm platter and top each plate with the bacon, spinach, and slices of avocado. Add the egg on top.
5. Serve hot.

Baked Eggs in Avocado

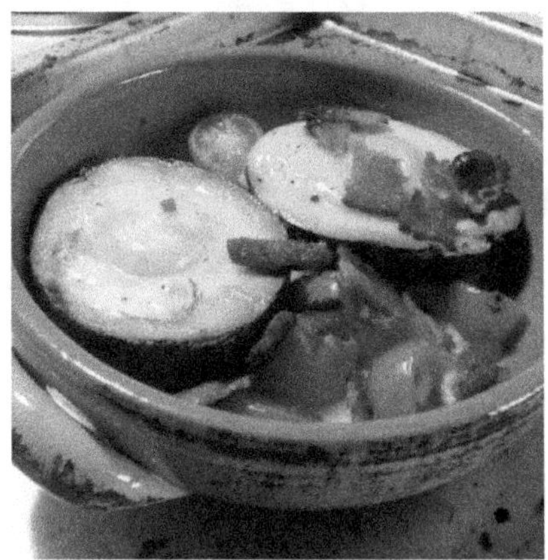

2 servings
Macronutrients: 8 g Protein | 23 g Fats | 9 g Carbs|2 g Net Carbs

Ingredients:
- 2 eggs
- 1 ripened avocado
- Optional: Hot sauce
- To Taste:
  -Freshly cracked black pepper
  -Pink Himalayan salt

Method:
1. Warm up the oven until it reaches 425°F.
2. Slice the avocado into half and remove the pit. Use an ice cream scoop to remove about 1-2 tablespoons of the fleshy insides. Arrange the halves in a small baking pan. Crack an egg into both halves and season with some pepper and salt.
3. Bake 15-20 minutes.
4. If you want to spice the eggs and avocado up a little bit; just add some keto-friendly hot sauce.

BLT Breakfast Salad

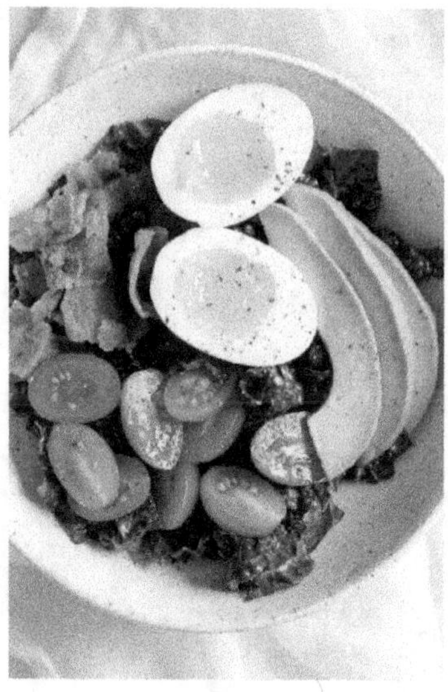

2 servings
Macronutrients: 18 g Protein|39 g Fats|18 g Carbs|4 g Net Carbs

Ingredients:
- 2 tbsp. olive oil
- 5 oz. mixed greens
- 2 large eggs
- 1 thinly sliced avocado
- To Taste:
  -Freshly cracked black pepper
  -Pink Himalayan salt
- 5 grape tomatoes – halved
- 6 cooked and chopped bacon slices

Method:
1. Prepare a saucepan of water using the high heat setting. When it starts to boil, gently add the eggs and lower to med-high. Cook for 6 minutes.

2. Meanwhile, toss the oil and greens into two bowls and add the salt and pepper.
3. Prepare the salad with the tomatoes, avocado slices, and bacon bits.
4. When the eggs are done, peel and slice into halves for each of the salads. Serve and enjoy or store in the fridge.

Brussels Sprouts, Eggs & Bacon for Brunch

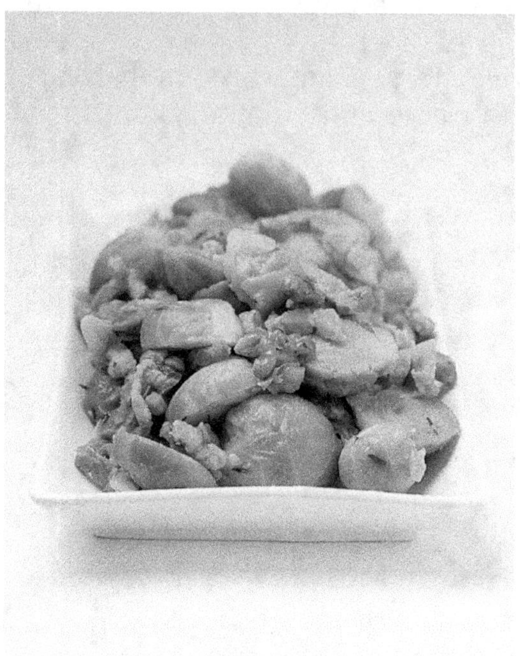

2 servings
Macronutrients: 27 g Protein | 29 g Fats | 12 g Carbs| 7 g Net Carbs

Ingredients:
- 1 tbsp. olive oil
- 4 large eggs
- 1/2 lb. Brussels sprouts
- 6 slices diced bacon
- 2 tbsp. grated parmesan cheese
- Black pepper & Pink salt – to taste

- Also Needed: 9x13-inch baking pan

Method:
1. Clean trim and slice the sprouts into halves. Warm up the oven to 400°F.

2. Toss the sprouts into the oil, salt, and pepper.
3. Lightly spray the baking pan with cooking spray. Arrange the bacon and sprouts in the pan. Roast them until they are done (12 min.).
4. Transfer it to the stovetop and stir. Create four wells in the center and break the four eggs into each one.
5. Sprinkle the eggs with the pepper, salt, and red pepper flakes. Sprinkle with the cheese. Roast for 8 more minutes.
6. Garnish with some nuts but add the carbs.

Cheesy Egg & Spinach Nest

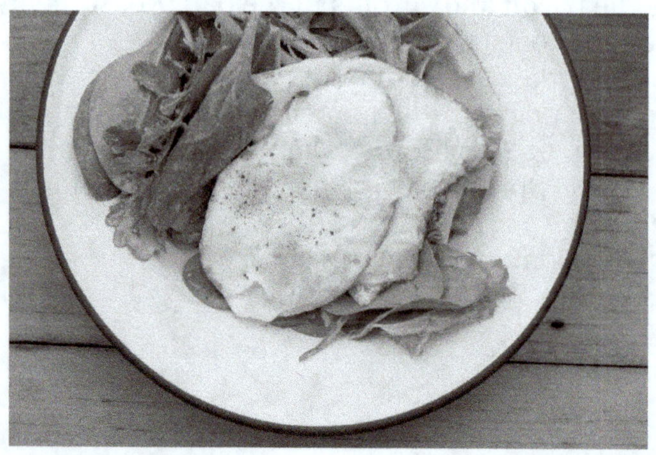

1 serving
Macronutrients: 31 g Protein |46 g Fats |9 g Carbs| 4 g Net Carbs

Ingredients:
- 1 tbsp. olive oil
- 2 large eggs
- 1/2 cup mozzarella cheese
- To Taste:
  -Freshly cracked black pepper
  -Pink Himalayan salt
- 1/2 diced avocado
- 1/4 cup spinach
- 1 tbsp. parmesan

Method:
1. Do the Prep: Use a handheld box grater to shred the parmesan and mozzarella. Tear apart the spinach, and dice the avocado.
2. Warm up the oil in a skillet using the med-high setting. Once hot, add the two eggs, salt, and pepper.

3. The edges will set after about 2 minutes. Sprinkle with part of the cheese and add the avocado and spinach to make a nest.
4. Cook until the cheese is browned and crispy (7-10 min.).
5. Serve on a warm plate and enjoy.

Cheesy Muffins

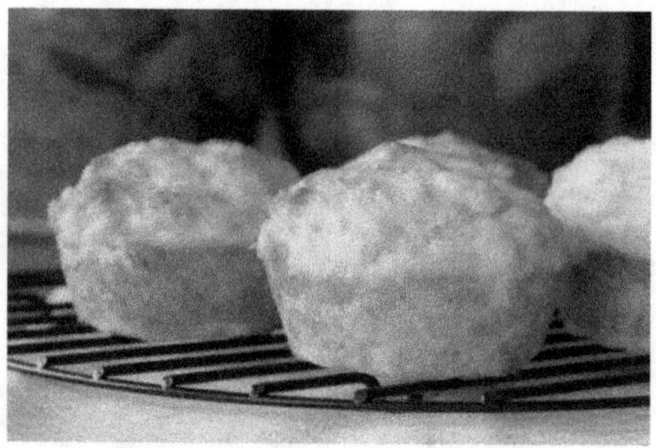

12 servings
Macronutrients: 13.7 g Protein | 39.9 g Fats | 5.5 Carbs| 4.3 Net Carbs

Ingredients:
- 1/2 tsp. of each:
  -Baking soda
  -Dried thyme
- 1/4 tsp. salt
- 2 cups almond flour
- 1/8 cup melted butter
- 1 cup of each:
  -Sour cream
  -Colby jack cheese
- 2 eggs
- 1/2 cup shredded muenster cheese

Method:
1. Warm up the oven to 400°F. Prepare the muffin tin with cupcake liners.
2. Whisk the dry fixings in one container.
3. In another dish, whisk the eggs, sour cream, and butter. Stir in the egg, and lastly, the flour mix. Tip: If it's too thin, add 1 tbsp. of heavy cream or water.
4. Fold in the cheese and mix. Spoon into the pan – filling about three-quarters of the way to the tops.

5. Bake for five minutes and lower the heat to 350°F for 20 additional minutes.
6. Cool and serve.

Coconut Flour – Cream Cheese Pancakes

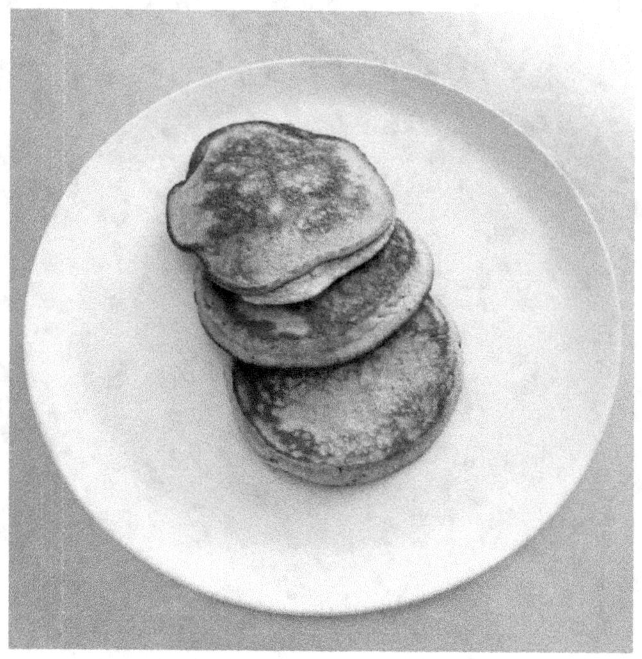

2 servings
Macronutrients: 9 g Protein |21 g Fats | 7 g Carbs| 4 g Net Carbs

Ingredients:
- 2 oz. softened cream cheese
- 2 large eggs
- 3 tbsp. coconut flour
- 2 tbsp. heavy cream/your choice milk
- 1 tbsp. sweetener – ex. erythritol
- 1/2 tsp. of each:
  -Optional – vanilla extract
  -Baking powder

Method:
1. Puree all of the fixings in a blender until creamy. Wait for the batter to thicken for 2 minutes.

2. Fry 4 (3-inch) pancakes for 1-2 minutes per side. They're ready when the bubbles form on the edges.
3. Serve and enjoy with your favorite keto-friendly toppings.

Kale – Avocado & Egg Skillet

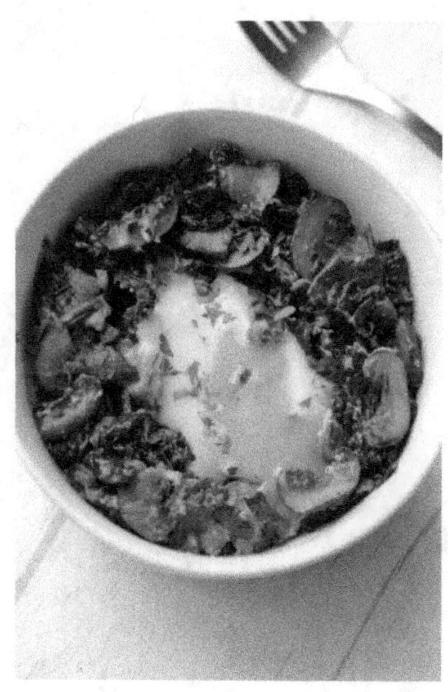

2 servings

Macronutrients: 18 g Protein| 34 g Fats |13 g Carbs|6 g Net Carbs

Ingredients:
- 2 tbsp. olive oil – divided
- 1 sliced avocado
- 5 oz. fresh kale
- 2 cups sliced mushrooms
- 4 large eggs
- To Taste:
  -Freshly cracked black pepper
  -Pink Himalayan salt

Method:
1. Warm up a skillet on the stovetop with 1 tablespoon of the oil.
2. When it's hot, toss in the mushrooms and saute for three minutes.

3. Shred the kale into ribbons. Use the rest of the oil to massage the kale (1-2 min).
4. Add to the skillet with the mushrooms and lastly, add the avocado (or serve it on the side).
5. Create four wells in the mixture using a spoon. Add an egg and flavor to your liking. Cover the pan for about 5 minutes or until the eggs are done to your liking.

Perfect Scrambled Eggs

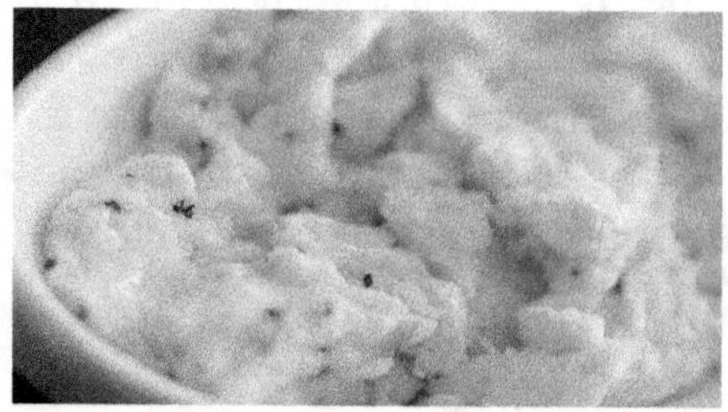

2 servings
Macronutrients: 11 g Protein | 15 g Fats | 1 g Carbs| 1 g Net Carbs

Ingredients:
- 1-2 tbsp water
- 4 eggs
- 1 tbsp. butter
- To Taste
  - Ground black pepper
  - Salt
- Optional Topping: Freshly chopped chives or sliced scallion – green parts

Method:
1. Crack the eggs and add the water into a mixing bowl. Whisk until well mixed.
2. Use the med-high heat setting on the stovetop to warm a skillet. Add the butter. When melted, scramble the eggs with a quick swirl. Lower the heat to medium and continue scrambling the eggs making sure to keep the 'raw' eggs in contact with the pan until done (3-4 min.). Reduce the temperature to low until entirely done. Sprinkle with the salt and pepper.
3. Serve with your chosen topping.

11.2. Beverages

Bulletproof Coffee

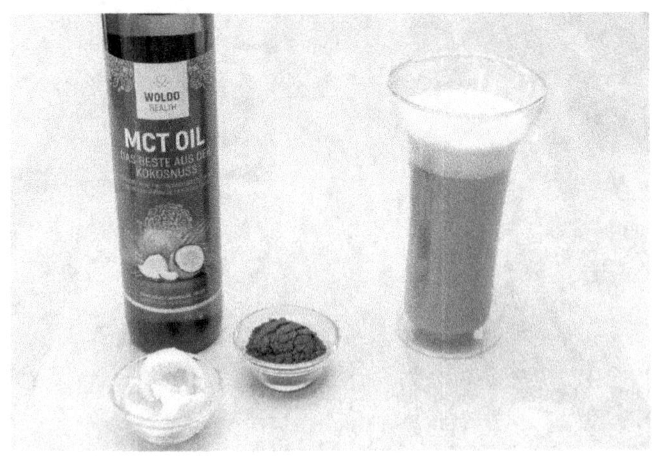

1 serving
Macronutrients: 1 g Protein | 51 g Fats | -0- g Carbs| -0- g
Net Carbs

Ingredients:

- 2 tbsp. of each:
  -MCT oil powder
  -Ghee/butter
- 1 1/2 c. hot coffee

Method:
1. Empty the hot coffee into your blender.
2. Pour in the powder and butter. Blend until frothy.
3. Enjoy using a large mug.

11.3. Bread

Keto Bread

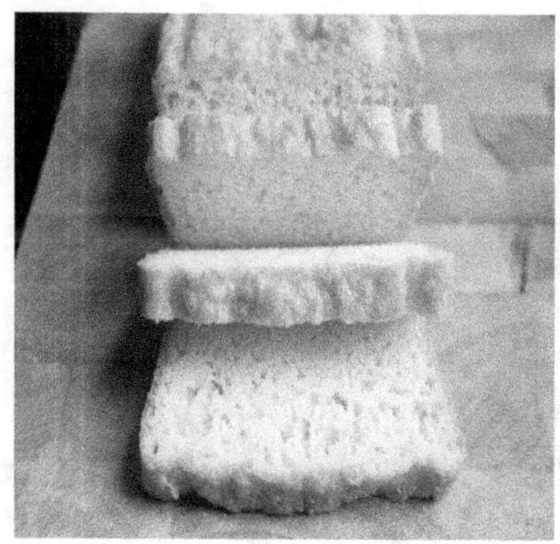

1 Loaf – 12 servings
Macronutrients: 6 g Protein |15 g Fats |4 g Carbs| 2 g Net Carbs

Ingredients:
- 5 tbsp. room temperature butter – divided
- Optional: 1 scoop MCT oil powder – ex Perfect Keto
- 3 tsp. baking powder
- 1.5 cups almond flour
- 1 pinch of salt
- 6 large eggs

- Also Needed: 5x9-inch loaf pan

Method:
1. Warm up the oven until it reaches 390°F. Grease the pan with 1 tablespoon of butter.
2. Use a hand mixer to combine the flour, rest of the butter, the baking powder, salt, eggs, and MCT powder (if using) in a large mixing container.

3. Mix well and empty into the prepared pan.
4. Bake until nicely browned (25 min.). Slice and serve.

90-Second Bread-In-A-Mug

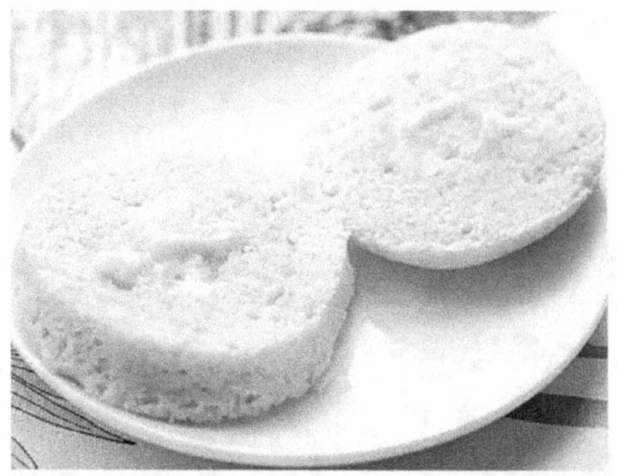

1 serving
Macronutrients: 14.5 g Protein |36.4 g Fats |9.8 g Carbs| 5.4 g Net Carbs

Ingredients:
- 1 tbsp. butter
- 1/3 cup blanched almond flour
- 1 pinch salt
- 1/2 tsp. baking powder
- 1 egg

Method:
1. Prepare a microwave-safe mug with the butter. Melt 15 seconds.
2. Swirl the butter around the mug.
3. Whisk the dry fixings and pour into the mug.
4. Cook for about 90 seconds and let cool for 2 minutes.
5. Turn the mug upside down, and it should easily slide out for slicing. If not, use a sharp knife to take it out.

11.4. Lunchtime Delights

Alfredo Pizza

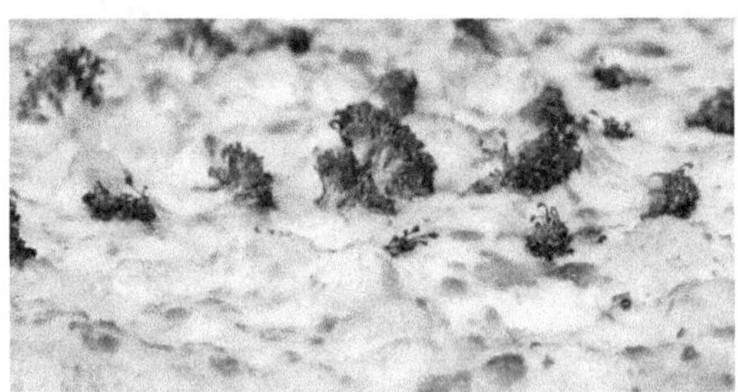

8 servings
Macronutrients: 9.5 g Protein |11.9 g Fats | 2.8g Carbs| 2.8 g
Net Carbs

Ingredients:
- 1 tbsp. organic roasted garlic & olive oil
- 2 tbsp. ghee
- 1 cup of each:
  -Shredded mozzarella
  -Pizza shredded cheese blend
- 1/4 cup mascarpone cheese
- 1 tbsp. heavy cream
- 1/8 tsp. lemon pepper
- 2 pinches salt
- 1/3 c. steamed broccoli
- 1 tsp. minced garlic
- 1/8 cup or 1 oz. Asiago cheese

Method:
1. Using the medium heat setting, warm up the oil in a skillet.
2. Add the pizza cheese once it's hot. Form a circle as the pizza dough.

3. Add the mozzarella and continue to simmer 4-5 minutes. When it's crispy, set aside in a plate to cool.
4. Using the same pan, cook the mascarpone, cream, salt, ghee, lemon pepper, and garlic. Simmer to bubbling.
5. Steam the broccoli according to the package instructions. Drain well.
6. Arrange the rest of the fixings over the 'crust' adding the broccoli and asiago last.

Bacon Stir Fry for Brunch

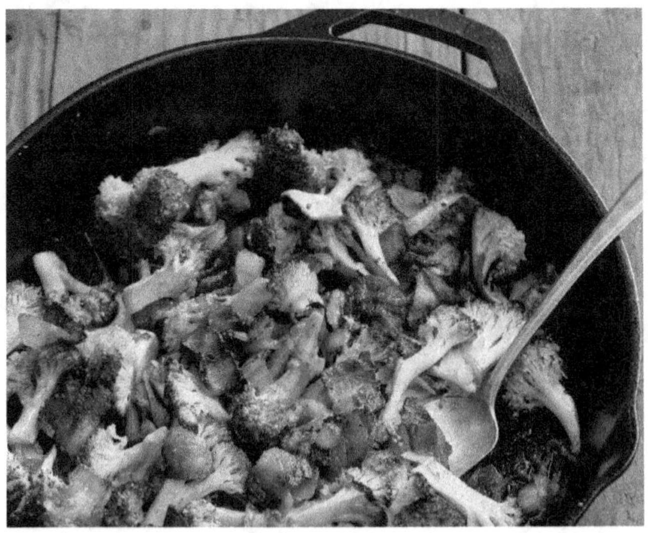

3 servings
Macronutrients: 10.5 g Protein | 15.6 g Fats |17.9 g Carbs|
8.6 g Net Carbs

Ingredients:
- 5 strips of bacon
- 1 tbsp. keto-friendly soy sauce
- 3 c. frozen –mixed veggies or broccoli

Method:

1. Slice the bacon into small bits. Prepare over high heat in a skillet.
2. Toss in the veggies and stir-fry until softened.
3. Sprinkle in the sauce, toss, and serve.

Broccoli & Cheese Soup

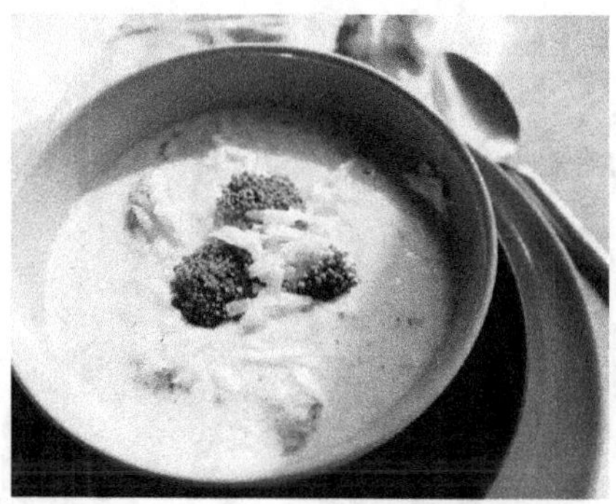

4 servings

Macronutrients: 10 g Protein | 37 g Fats |4 g Carbs|3 g Net Carbs

Ingredients:
- 2 tbsp. butter
- To Taste:
  -Freshly cracked black pepper
  -Pink Himalayan salt
- 1 cup of each:
  -Vegetable or chicken broth
  -Heavy whipping cream
  -Finely chopped broccoli florets
  -Sharp shredded cheese – divided

Method:
1. Melt the butter in a saucepan over medium heat. Break apart the broccoli and add to the pan to saute for 5 minutes.
2. Stir in the broth and cream with a shake of salt and pepper.
3. Continue - occasionally stirring for 10-15 more minutes.
4. Once it's thickened, reduce the heat to the low temperature and slowly add the shredded cheese – saving a little for garnishing the bowls of soup.

5. Portion into four bowls and enjoy.

Carnitas - Crockpot

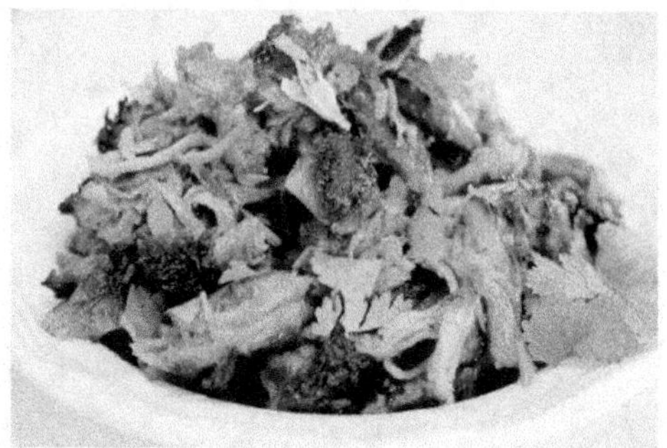

2 servings
Macronutrients: 45 g Protein | 26 g Fats |6 g Carbs|4 g Net Carbs

Ingredients:
- 1 lb. boneless pork butt roast
- 1/2 tbsp. chili powder
- 1 tbsp. olive oil
- 1/2 small diced onion
- 2 minced cloves of garlic
- Juice of 1 lime
- To Taste:
  -Freshly cracked black pepper
  -Pink Himalayan salt

Method:
1. Use the low-temperature setting to warm up the crockpot.
2. Whisk the olive oil with the chili powder. Rub over the pork and place in the cooker – the fatty side facing up.
3. Prepare the veggies and add along with the lime juice, salt, and pepper.
4. Place the lid on the pot and simmer on low for 8 hours. After that time, you can brown it in a warm oven to crisp it up if desired (350°F).

5. When ready, shred the meat on a cutting board using two forks.
6. Enjoy on a leaf of lettuce, but remember to add any additional carbs.

Crockpot Chicken Chowder

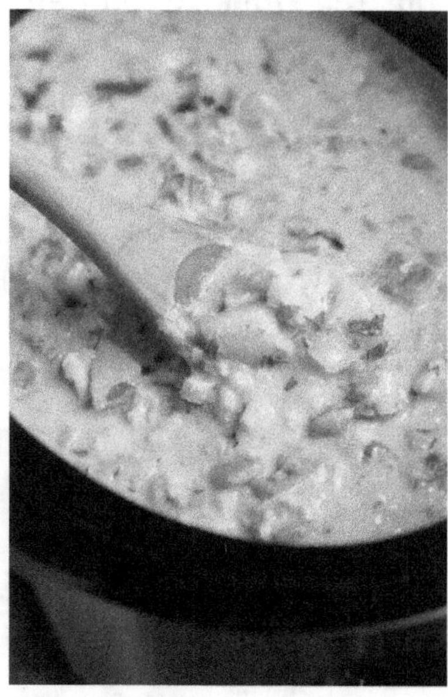

4 servings
Macronutrients: 39.7 g Protein |28.8 g Fats |9.7 g Carbs| 7.5 g Net Carbs

Ingredients:
- 1 lb. chicken breasts – skinless & boneless
- 14 oz. diced tomatoes
- 1 small onion
- 0.5 oz. diced jalapeno
- 1 cup chicken broth
- 8 oz. cream cheese
- 1.6 oz lime juice
- 1 garlic clove
- 1 tbsp. of each:
  -Black pepper
  -Cilantro
- 1 tsp. salt

Method:

1. Chop the garlic and cilantro. Dice the onion and jalapeno.
2. Combine all of the fixings in the crockpot. Prepare using the low-temperature setting for 6-9 hours or high for 4 hours.
3. Once it is done, shred the chicken in the pot using 2 forks.
4. Serve and enjoy.
5. Note: For variations, just add different veggies to the mix, but remember to add the carbs.

Cucumber Sandwich

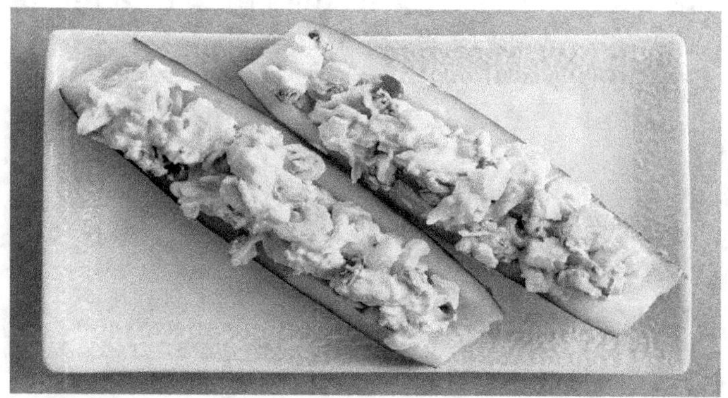

1 serving

Macronutrients: 30.1 g Protein | 18.5 g Fats | 15.3 g Carbs| 12.6 g Net Carbs

Ingredients:
- 2 tbsp. pesto
- 1/4 chopped red pepper
- 1 cucumber
- 1/2 c. shredded cooked chicken
- 0.5 oz shredded parmesan cheese
- For Extra Flavor: Pepper and Salt

Method:
1. Combine all of the fixings in a mixing container – omitting the cucumber.
2. Slice the cucumber in half and carefully remove the core (as shown in the picture).
3. Add the goodies to the scooped portion and enjoy your sandwich.

Pizza Bites

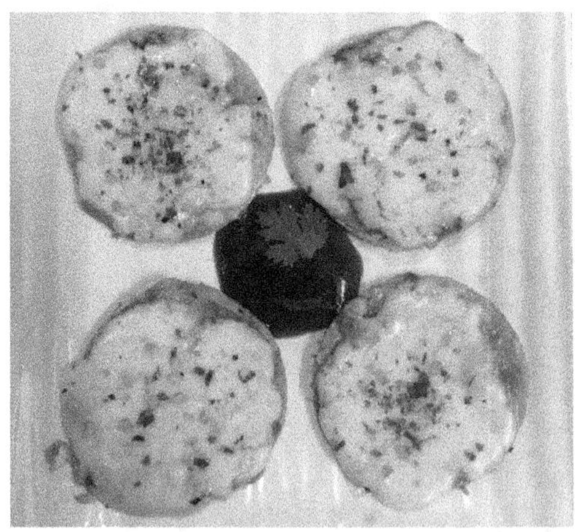

4 servings
Macronutrients: 5.2 g Protein |6.8 g Fats |2.8 g Carbs| 2.8 g Net Carbs

Ingredients:
- 4 slices of salami
- 1/4 cup of each:
  -Marinara sauce
  -Shredded mozzarella

Method:
1. Warm up the broiler using the oven (high setting). Add the salami on a baking sheet.
2. Sprinkle with the sauce and cheese.
3. Prepare in the oven for 5 minutes.
4. Let them drain the grease on a towel for 1 to 2 minutes. Serve.

11.5. Salads

Chicken Salad

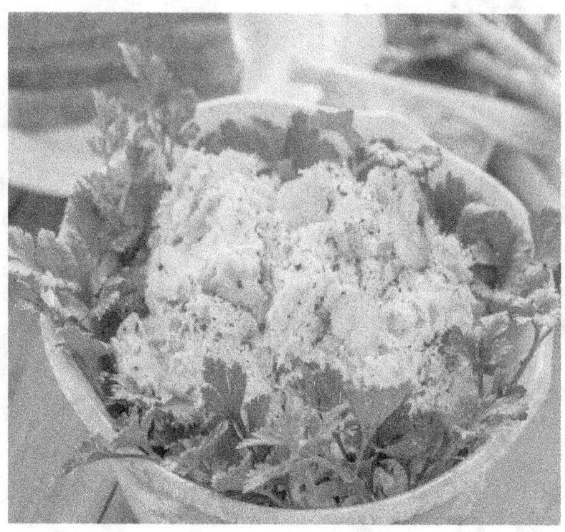

3 servings
Macronutrients: 17.6 g Protein | 12 g Fats | 8 g Carbs| 8 g
Net Carbs

Ingredients:

- 1 stalk 11-12-inches
- 1 green onion
- 2 tbsp. parsley
- 1 hard-boiled egg
- 5 oz. roasted chicken breast
- 1/3 cup mayonnaise
- 1/8 tsp. granulated garlic
- 1/2 tbsp. relish
- 1 tsp. Dijon mustard
- Pepper & Salt – if desired

Method:
1. Mince the chicken and boiled egg.

2. You can dice and toss all of the veggies into a food processor. Pulse until they're the desired consistency. Next, throw in the chicken and blend. Add to a dish and do the same with the egg.
3. Add all of the fixings and season to your liking. Serve any time.

Chopped Greek Salad

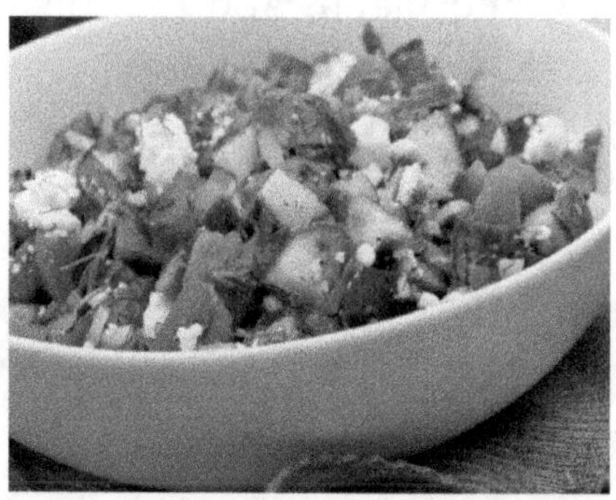

2 servings
Macronutrients: 4 g Protein |19 g Fats |4 g Carbs|2 g Net Carbs

Ingredients:
- 1/2 cup halved grape tomatoes
- 2 cups chopped romaine
- 1/4 cup of each:
  -Kalamata black olives
  -Crumbled feta cheese
- 2 tbsp vinaigrette dressing
- 1 tbsp. olive oil
- Pink salt and Pepper to taste

Method:
1. Prepare the salad with the romaine as a base. Build it your way and give it a drizzle of the oil and vinegar.
2. Serve in two salad dishes and enjoy.

Salmon & Caesar Salad

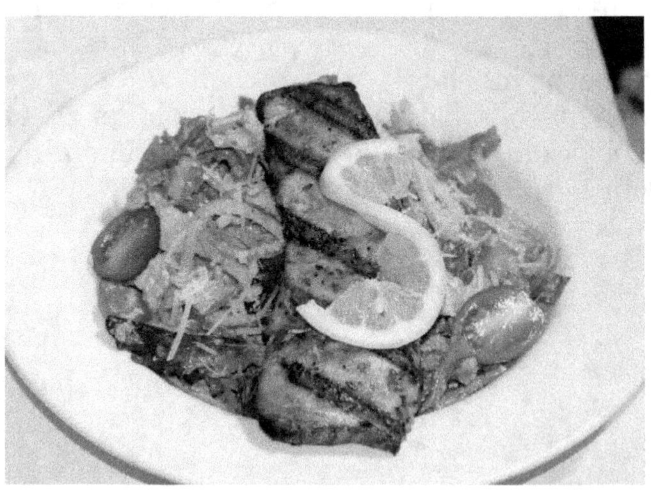

2 servings
Macronutrients: 40 g Protein | 32 g Fats |6 g Carbs|2 g Net Carbs

Ingredients:
- 2 salmon fillets – 6 oz. ea.
- 4 slices of bacon
- 1 tbsp. ghee – if needed
- Pinch of each:
  -Freshly ground black pepper
  -Pink salt
- 1/2 sliced avocado
- 2 cups chopped romaine or 2 romaine hearts
- 2 tbsp. Caesar dressing

Method:
1. Cook the bacon until crispy for 8 minutes using the med-high heat setting on the stovetop. Drain on a platter using paper towels.
2. Remove the excess water from the fillets. Give them a shake of pepper and salt.

3. Use the same pan to prepare the salmon. Add butter if needed.
4. Cook for five minutes per side. This will be medium-rare.
5. Break the bacon into bits.
6. Prepare the two salad dishes with equal parts of romaine, avocado, and the bacon. Add the salmon.
7. Enjoy with a drizzle of the dressing and enjoy!

Shrimp & Avocado Salad

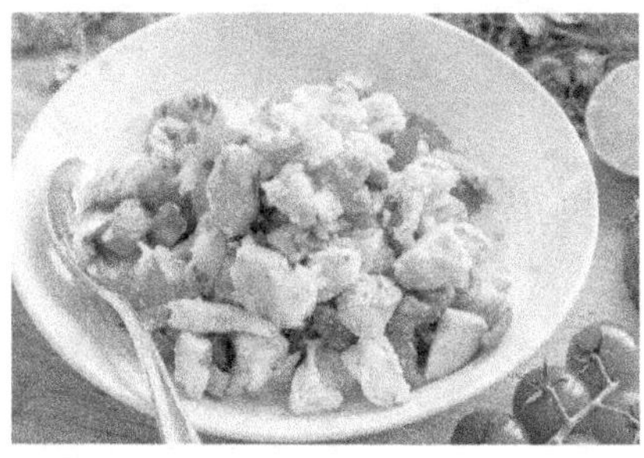

2 servings
Macronutrients: 50 g Protein | 41 g Fats |8 g Carbs| 3 g Net Carbs

Ingredients:
- 1 lb. med. cooked shrimp
- 1 tbsp. olive oil
- 1 cubed avocado
- 1/4 cup mayonnaise
- To Taste:
  -Freshly cracked black pepper
  -Pink Himalayan salt
- 1 chopped celery stalk
- 1 tsp. lime juice – 1 lime

Method:
1. Squeeze the lime to get one teaspoon of juice.
2. Remove the tail, devein, and peel the shrimp. Give it a shake of salt and pepper.
3. Warm up a skillet (med. heat) and pour in the oil. Once it gets hot, toss the shrimp and cook until they are pink (1-2 min.). Take from the burner so the shrimp will cool. Place in a closed container and put in the refrigerator.
4. In a mixing container, combine the mayo, celery, and avocado. Stir in the juice and more salt if desired. Combine all of the fixings with the cold shrimp.

5. Refrigerate the salad for at least 30 minutes before
   serving.

Tomato – Avocado & Cucumber Salad

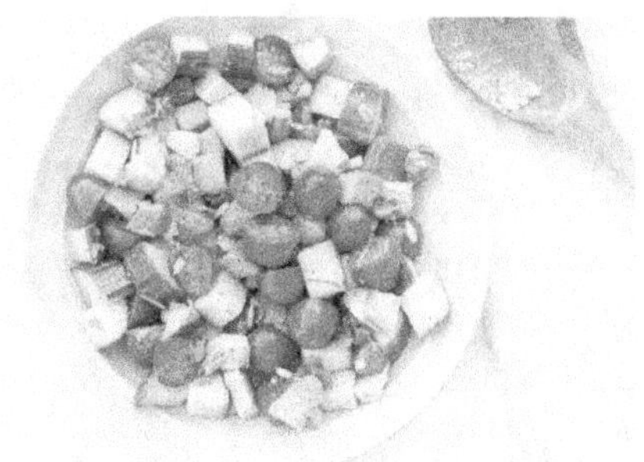

2 servings
Macronutrients: 5 g Protein |23 g Fats |12 g Carbs|6 g Net
Carbs

Ingredients:
- 1 English cucumber
- 1 avocado
- 1/2 cup halved grape tomatoes
- 2 tbsp. vinaigrette salad dressing
- To Taste:
  -Freshly cracked black pepper
  -Pink Himalayan salt
- 1/4 cup crumbled feta cheese

Method:
1. Finely chop the cucumber and avocado. Cut the tomatoes into halves. Combine the veggies and crumbled feta cheese.
2. Spritz with the vinaigrette and sprinkle with the salt and pepper.
3. Toss and divide into two portions. Serve and enjoy.

11.6. Dinner Specialties

Beef Short Ribs

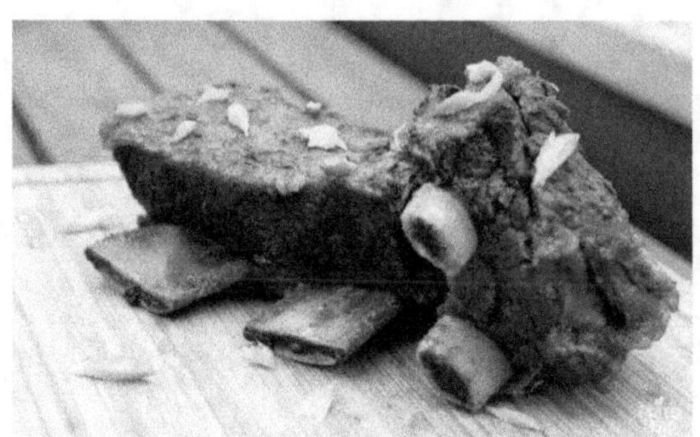

4 servings
Macronutrients: 25.7 g Protein | 62 g Fats | 2.5 g Carbs| 2.5 g Net Carbs

Ingredients:
- 1/4 cup keto-friendly soy sauce
- 6 (4-oz) beef short ribs
- 2 tbsp. of each:
  -Fish sauce
  -Rice vinegar
- 1/4 tsp. cardamom
- 1 tbsp. salt
- 1 tsp. ground ginger
- 1/2 tsp. of each:
  -Minced garlic
  -Sesame seeds
  -Red pepper flakes
  -Onion powder

Method:
1. Mix the fish sauce, vinegar, and alternative soy sauce.
2. Arrange the ribs in a dish with high sides. Add the sauce and marinade for up to 1 hour.

3. Combine all of the spices together. Take the ribs from the dish and sprinkle with the rub.
4. Warm up the grill (med-high) and cook for 3-5 minutes per side. Serve and enjoy.

Buffalo Chicken Casserole

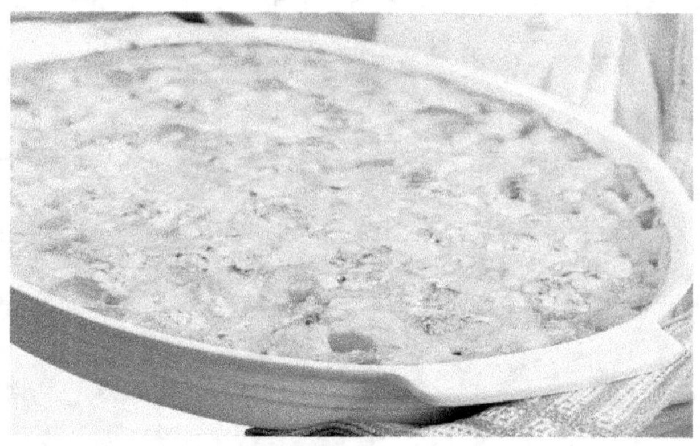

6 servings
Macronutrients: 54.6 g Protein | 43.9 g Fats |5.1 g Carbs| 5.1 g Net Carbs

Ingredients:
- 1.85 lb. chicken thighs
- 1.25 lb. bacon
- 1.5 oz. jalapenos
- 4 oz. cheddar cheese
- 2 oz. mozzarella cheese
- 1/4 c. of each:
  -Mayonnaise
  -Hot sauce
- To Taste:
  -Freshly cracked black pepper
  -Pink Himalayan salt

Method:
1. Warm up the oven until it reaches 400°F.
2. Discard all of the bones and sprinkle the chicken with the pepper and salt.
3. Cover a baking pan with foil and arrange a wire rack on top of that to place the chicken. Cook for 40 minutes.

4. Chop the bacon to bits and fry in a skillet until crispy using the medium heat setting on the stovetop. Add the jalapenos once it's almost done. When they're softened, stir in the hot sauce and cream cheese. Mix well.
5. When done, transfer the chicken to the countertop to cool. Remove the skin and cover with the cream mixture. Bake 10-15 minutes. Broil on high for 3-5 minutes.
6. Let it cool down for about 5 minutes and serve.

Bun-less Bacon Burgers

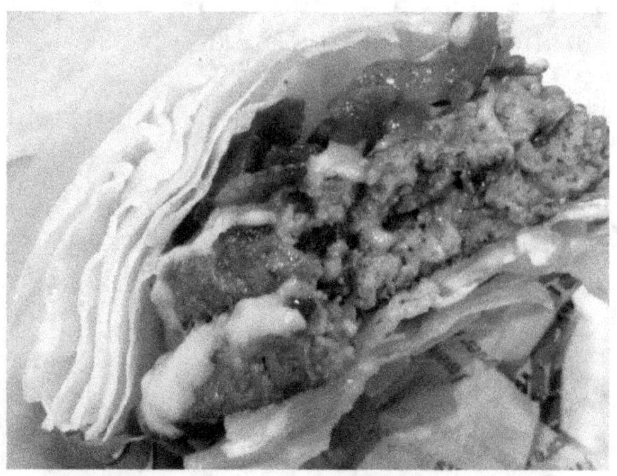

4 servings
Macronutrients: 58.9 g Protein | 19.7 g Fats| 2.9 g Carbs| 2.2 g Net Carbs

Ingredients:
- 8 leaves romaine lettuce
- 1 1/2 lb. ground beef
- 3.95 oz. pepper jack cheese
- 1 onion
- Salt and Pepper to taste

Method:
1. Shape the beef into four patties (or make 8 to double like the one in the picture – same carbs). Prepare using the medium heat setting in a skillet. Cook until well-done throughout. Fry the bacon in the same pan. Drain both on a paper-lined platter.
2. Use the lettuce leaves as a bun and season to your liking. Melt the cheese onto the patties and serve on the romaine.

Cheesy Steak

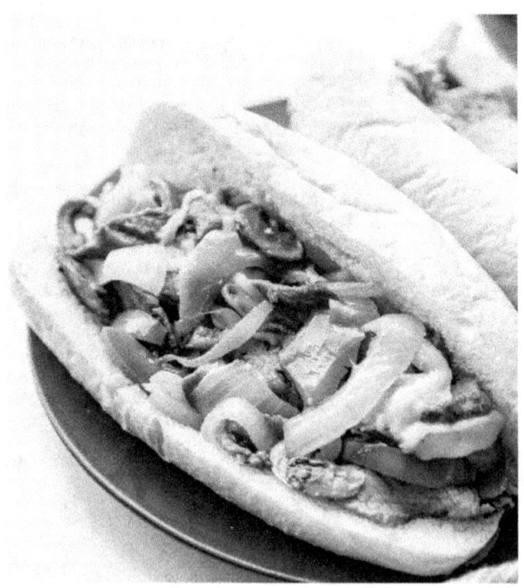

2 servings

Macronutrients: 53.3 g Protein | 53.5 g Fats |10.5 g Carbs|9.6 g Net Carbs

Ingredients:

- 1 tbsp. of each:
  -Olive oil
  -Ghee
  -Dijon mustard
  -Minced garlic
- 1 lb. shaved beef steak
- 1/4 cup – chopped of each:
  -Green peppers
  -Onions
- 2 tbsp. mayonnaise
- 4 slices American cheese
- 4 keto bread slices

Method:

1. On the med-low setting on the stovetop, add the ghee. When hot, add the peppers, onions, and garlic along with the olive oil.
2. Slice the steak to 1/8-inch thickness (as shown in the picture). Add when the oil is hot.
3. Brown the steak and lower the temperature to the low setting.
4. Combine the Dijon and mayo. Add the cheese to the steak for 1 minute. Combing the fixings.
5. Put it in between two keto bread slices or enjoy it alone without the bread.

Chuck Steak – Slow Cooker

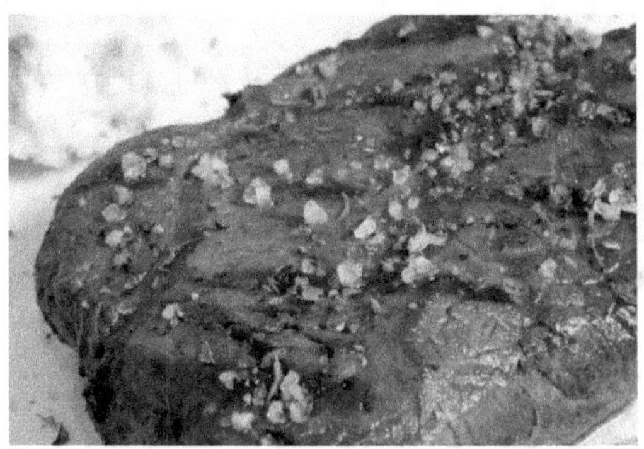

8 servings
Macronutrients: 78.5 g Protein | 32.8 g Fats | 3.6 g Carbs|
2.9 g Net Carbs

Ingredients:
- 1 (4.4 lb.) chuck steak
- 4 celery stalks
- 3 carrots
- 2 garlic cloves
- 2 cups beef stock
- 1 cup red wine
- Optional: 1/4 cup diced onion – add any carbs
- Salt and Pepper to taste

Method:
1. Pour 1 inch of water into the cooker. Add the roast and prepare on the high setting for 4 hours.
2. Slice the veggies and toss them around the roast.
3. Empty the wine and broth over the meat and add all of the spices.
4. Simmer four more hours on the high setting and enjoy.
5. Slice the steak into 8 servings and serve with the veggies.

Coconut Shrimp

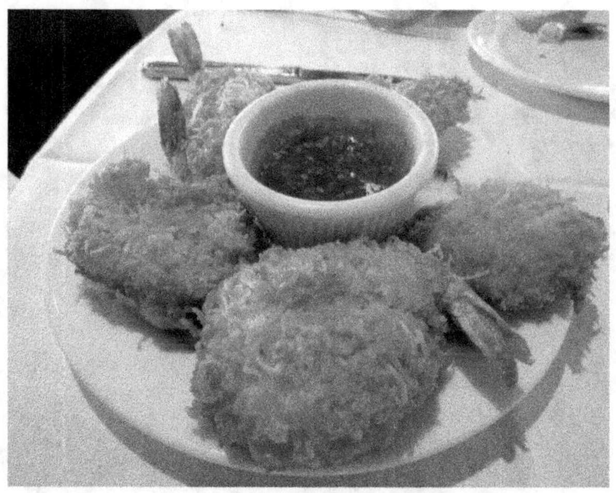

3 servings
Macronutrients: 38 g Protein | 36.4 g Fats | 13.8 **g** Carbs| 1.1 g Net Carbs

Ingredients:
- 1 lb. frozen pre-cooked shrimp
- 1 cup unsweetened coconut flakes
- 2 large egg whites
- 2 tbsp. coconut flour

Method:
1. Warm up the oven to reach 350°F. Thaw the shrimp to room temperature.
2. Add the egg whites to a mixing bowl. Whip until peaks are formed.
3. In two containers, add the flour and coconut flakes.
4. Dip the shrimp into the flour, egg whites, and lastly the coconut.
5. Arrange the shrimp on a lightly greased baking pan.
6. Bake for 15 minutes. Change to broil on high for 3-5 minutes.

Feta-Stuffed Burgers

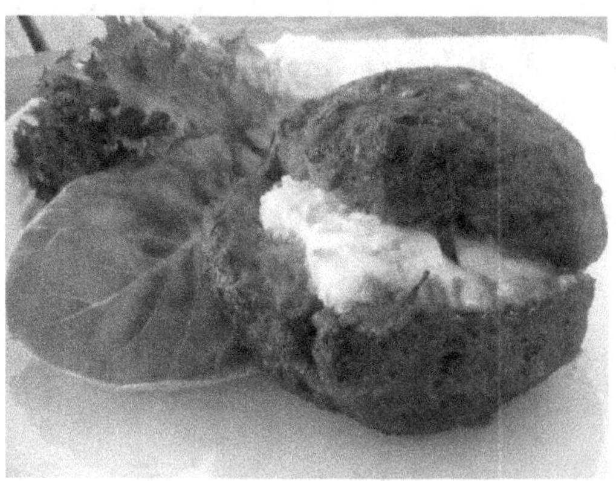

2 servings
Macronutrients: 41 g Protein | 48 g Fats | 2 g Carbs| 1 g Net
Carbs

Ingredients:

- 1 scallion
- 12 oz. pkg. ground beef & lamb
- 2 tbsp. chopped mint leaves
- 1 tbsp. of each:
  -Dijon mustard
  -Ghee
- 2 oz. crumbled feta cheese
- To Taste:
  -Freshly cracked black pepper
  -Pink Himalayan salt

Method:

1. Thinly slice the green and white parts of the scallion.
   Also, finely chop the fresh mint leaves. Crumble the
   feta.
2. Combine the mustard with the mint and scallions. Stir
   in the beef and lamb. Mix well and shape into four
   patties. Sprinkle with the salt and pepper.

3. Press feta cubes into two of the patties and place a
    patty on top (cheese in the middle). Seal it closed.
4. Using the medium heat setting, melt the ghee and add
    the patties once the pan is hot. Cook each side for 5
    minutes and serve.

Fried Pork Chops

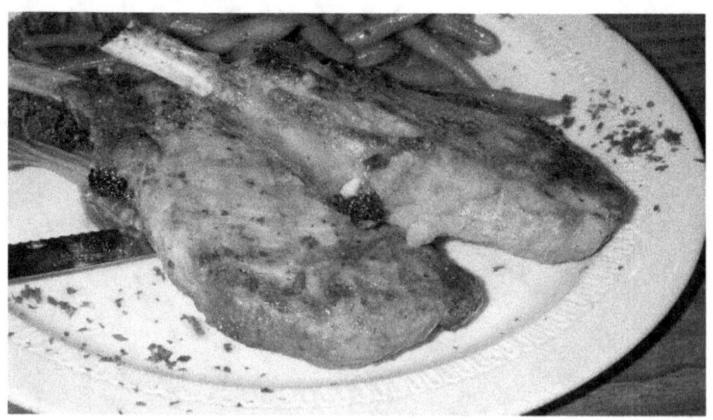

3 servings
Macronutrients: 22.1 g Protein | 27.1 g Fats | 12.4 g Carbs|
4.2 g Net Carbs

Ingredients:
- 1/2 cup coconut flour
- 3 pork chops
- 1 tsp. each:
  - Pepper
  - Salt
- 1 tbsp. butter

Method:
1. Combine all of the dry fixings in a large mixing container.
2. Pat the chops dry with a paper towel.
3. Melt the butter in a skillet on the stovetop.
4. Cover the chops with the mixture and prepare each side for 4-5 minutes.
5. Serve with your favorite side dishes.

Garlic Parmesan Wings

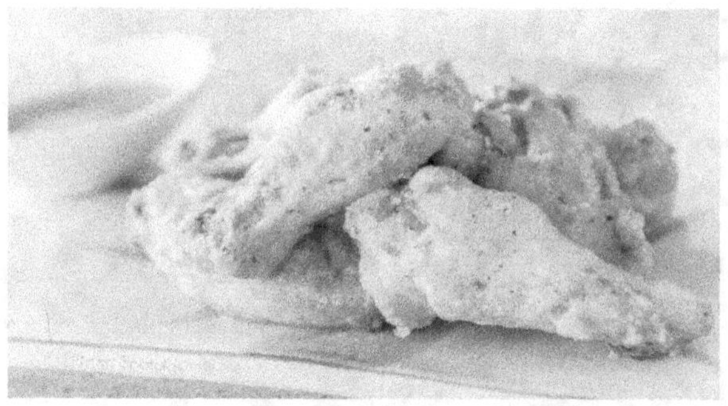

2 servings
Macronutrients: 23.6 g Protein |19.1 g Fats | 5.8 g Carbs| 5.3 g Net Carbs

Ingredients:

- 2 tbsp. garlic oil
- 1 tsp. garlic salt
- 2 individually frozen chicken wings
- 1/2 tbsp. garlic powder
- 1 oz. grated parmesan cheese

Method:

1. Warm up the oven to reach 450°F.
2. Add the wings to a baking pan and drizzle with the salt.
3. Bake for 35 minutes. Baste with part of the oil and broil for 5 minutes.
4. Once the skin is crispy, take it out of the oven, and add to a container with the rest of the oil, garlic powder, and parmesan cheese. Stir and serve.

Meatballs in the Crock

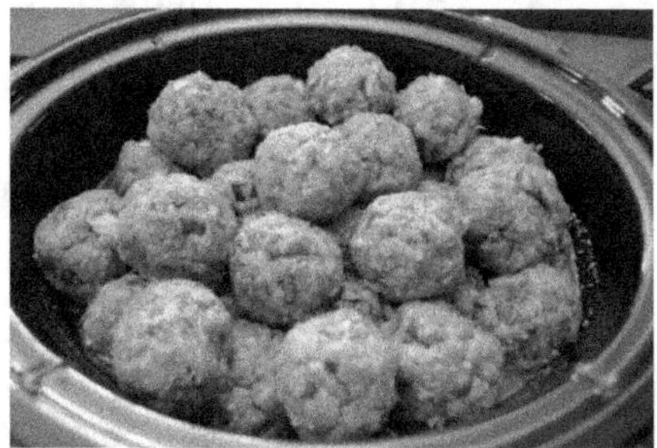

6 servings
Macronutrients: 49.2 g Protein|17.5 g Fats |5.7 g Carbs| 3.7 g
Net Carbs

Ingredients:
- 1 head of cauliflower
- 2 lb. ground beef
- 1 tbsp. cumin
- 1 tsp. paprika
- 2 heaping tbsp. tomato paste
- 2 cups bone broth
- Salt and Pepper to taste
- 1/4 cup of each:
  -Butter
  -Parsley

Method:
1. In a mixing dish, mix the meat with the salt, pepper, paprika, and cumin.
2. Shape into 1-inch meatballs and add to the crockpot. Make enough for 6 equal portions.
3. Mix the broth and tomato paste. Add to the pot and set the timer for 2 hours on the high setting or all day using the low heat setting.
4. Slice the cauliflower into florets and steak until softened – not mushy.

5. Drain away the water and add the salt, pepper, and butter. Add to a blender and mix until you have 'cauliflower' mashed potatoes. Add to a plate and serve with equal portions of meatballs.

Pork Kabobs

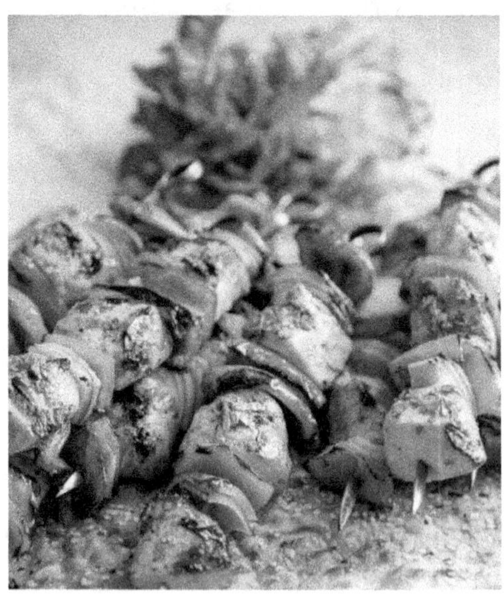

4 servings
Macronutrients: 33.7 g Protein | 8.6 g Fats | 5.5 g Carbs| 3.3 g Net Carbs

Ingredients:
- 2 tsp. hot sauce
- 3 tbsp sunflower seed butter
- 1 tbsp. of each:
  -Minced garlic
  -Keto-friendly soy sauce
  -Water
- 1/2 tsp. crushed red pepper
- 1 med. green pepper
- 1 lb. squared pork for kebabs
- Optional: Other Veggies – add the carbs

Method:
1. In a processor or blender, combine the water with the red pepper, soy sauce, garlic, butter, and hot sauce.

2. Slice the pork into squares. Cover with the marinade and rest for 1 hour.
3. Chop the peppers to fit the skewer. Thread the skewers alternating the pork and peppers.
4. Broil on high for 5 minutes per side.

Steak Pinwheels

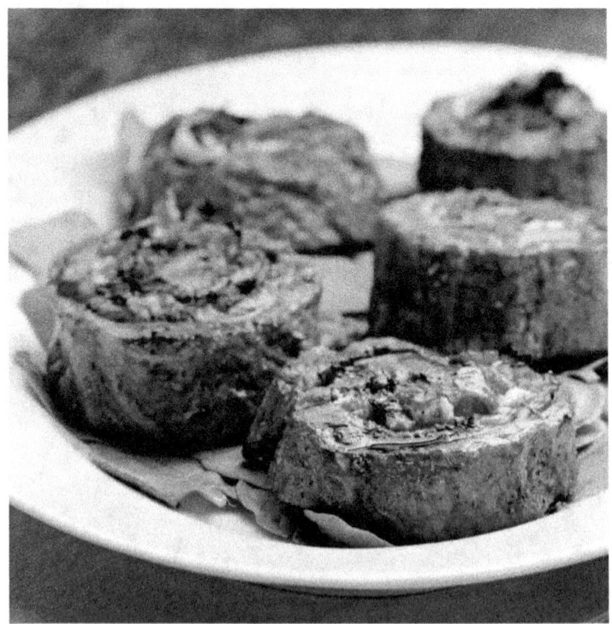

6 servings
Macronutrients: 54.5 g Protein | 19.5 g Fats | 3.4 g Carbs| 2.1 g Net Carbs

Ingredients:
- 2 lb. flank steak
- 1 pkg. (8 oz.) mozzarella cheese
- 1 bunch spinach – 1 3/4 cups approx.

Method:
1. Warm up the oven to 350°F.
2. Slice the steak into 6 portions and remove all of the 'hard' fat. Beat it thin with a mallet.
3. Shred the cheese with a food processor and sprinkle the steak. Roll it up and tie with a piece of cooking twine or a skewer.
4. Line the pan with the pinwheels and place on a layer of spinach.

5. Bake until done (25 min.).

11.7. Side Dishes

Baked Radishes & Brown Butter Sauce

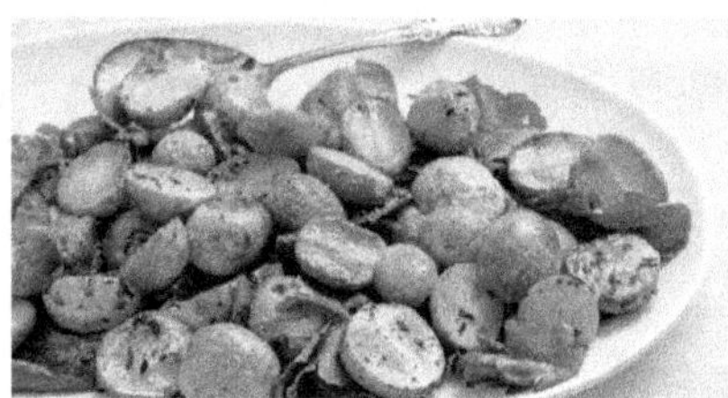

2 servings
Macronutrients: 1 g Protein |19 g Fats| 4 g Carbs |2 g Net Carbs

Ingredients:
- 2 cups halved radishes
- 1 tbsp. olive oil
- 2 tbsp. butter
- To Taste:
  -Freshly cracked black pepper
  -Pink Himalayan salt
- 1 tbsp. freshly chopped flat-leaf Italian parsley

Method:
1. Warm up the oven to reach 450°F.
2. Cut the radishes into halves and toss into the oil. Sprinkle with the pepper and salt.
3. Spread them on a baking tin – using a single layer. Bake in the preheated oven for 15 minutes. Stir about 1/2 way through the cycle.
4. After they have roasted 10 minutes, use the medium heat setting on the stovetop to melt the butter mixed with the salt. Simmer until it's a nutty brown (3 min.). Empty the butter into a mug and set aside.

5. Take the radishes out of the oven and portion into two
    plates. Add the butter and top it off with the fresh
    parsley to serve.

Baked Zucchini Gratin

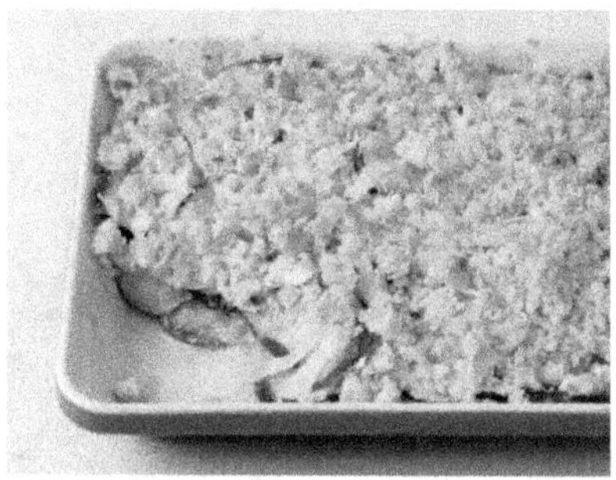

2 servings
Macronutrients: 28 g Protein |25 g Fats| 5 g Carbs|3 g Net Carbs

Ingredients:
- 1 oz. Brie cheese – rind removed
- 1 large zucchini – 1/4-inch slices
- 1/3 cup shredded Gruyere cheese
- 1 tbsp. butter
- To Taste:
  -Freshly cracked black pepper
  -Pink Himalayan salt
- 1/4 cup pork rinds

- Also Needed: 8-inch baking dish

Method:
1. Put the zucchini slices in a colander with the salt for 45 minutes.
2. Warm up the oven to reach 400°F.
3. After the zucchini has lost some of the juices (30 min.), heat the brie and butter in a small saucepan using the med-low setting. The process should take 2 minutes.
4. Arrange the zucchini in the baking dish – overlapping is okay. Give it a shake of pepper and add the brie mixture. Top it off with the gruyere cheese.

5. Lastly, add the crushed pork rinds and bake for 25 minutes. Once it's browned, serve and enjoy.

Buttery Mushrooms - Slow Cooked

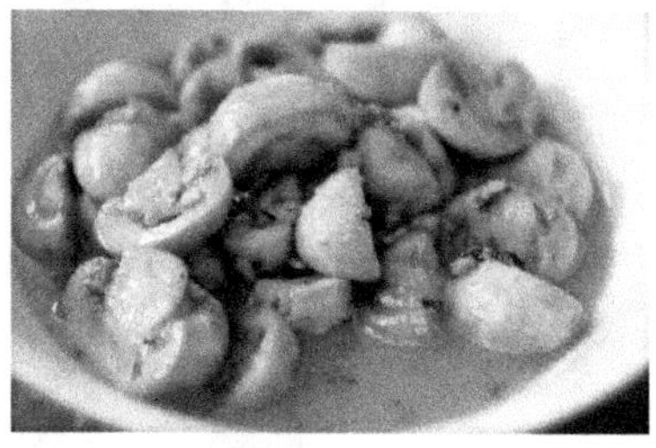

2 servings
Macronutrients: 28 g Protein |25 g Fats |5 g Carbs| 3 g Net
Carbs

Ingredients:
- 8 oz. fresh cremini mushrooms
- 1 tbsp. of each:
  -Pkg. dry ranch dressing mix
  -Freshly chopped flat-leaf Italian parsley
- 6 tbsp. butter
- 2 tbsp. grated parmesan cheese

Method:
1. Use the low setting to preheat the cooker with the insert in place.
2. Add the dry dressing with the butter. Stir well and add the mushrooms.
3. Sprinkle with the cheese and close the top.
4. Simmer for four hours on the low setting.
5. When ready, use a slotted spoon to serve the mushrooms.
6. Give it a sprinkle of the parsley and enjoy.

Cauliflower 'Potato' Salad - Vegetarian

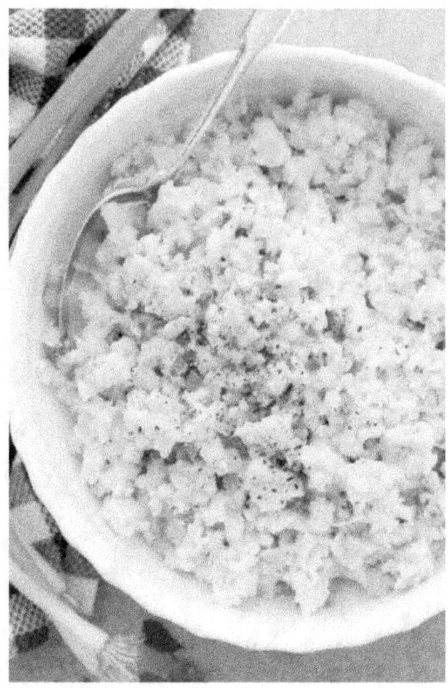

2 servings
Macronutrients: 5 g Protein |37 g Fats| 13 g Carbs| 8 g Net Carbs

Ingredients:
- 1 tbsp. of each:
  -Olive oil
  -Mustard – keto-friendly
- To Taste:
  -Freshly cracked black pepper
  -Pink Himalayan salt
- 1/2 head cauliflower
- 1/3 cup mayonnaise
- 1 tsp. paprika
- 1/4 cup dill pickles

Method:

1. Warm up the oven to 400°F. Prepare a cookie tin with a silicone baking mat or foil.

2. Dice the pickles and set aside. Slice the cauliflower into 1-inch pieces. Toss into a container with the oil, pepper, and salt.

3. Arrange it in the prepared pan and bake for 25 minutes. Toss it about halfway through the cooking cycle.

4. When done, combine with the mustard, pickles, and mayo. Shake with the paprika and chill in the fridge for 3 hours.

Parmesan & Pork Rind Green Beans

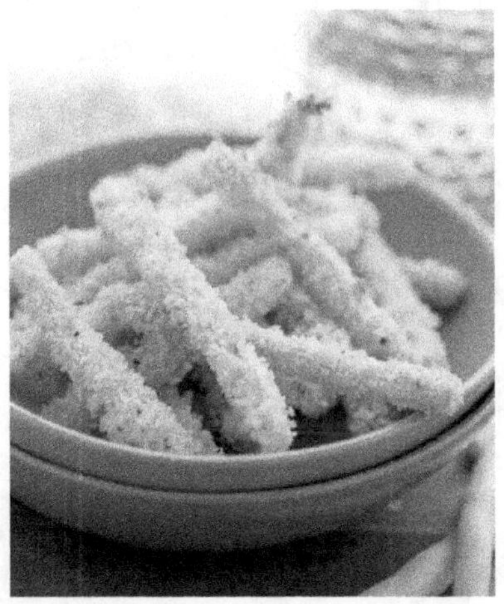

3 servings
Macronutrients: 6 g Protein |15 g Fats |8 g Carbs|5 g Net
Carbs

Ingredients:

- 1/2 lb. fresh green beans
- 2 tbsp. of each:
  -Olive oil
  -Crushed pork rinds
- 1 tbsp. grated parmesan cheese
- To Taste:
  -Freshly cracked black pepper
  -Pink Himalayan salt

Method:

1. Heat up the oven until it reaches 400°F.
2. Combine the oil with the beans, cheese, pepper, and salt. Toss well.
3. Arrange the mixture on the baking sheet and bake for 15 minutes.
4. Shake about halfway through the cooking cycle.
5. Portion the green beans and serve.

Vegetarian Deviled Eggs

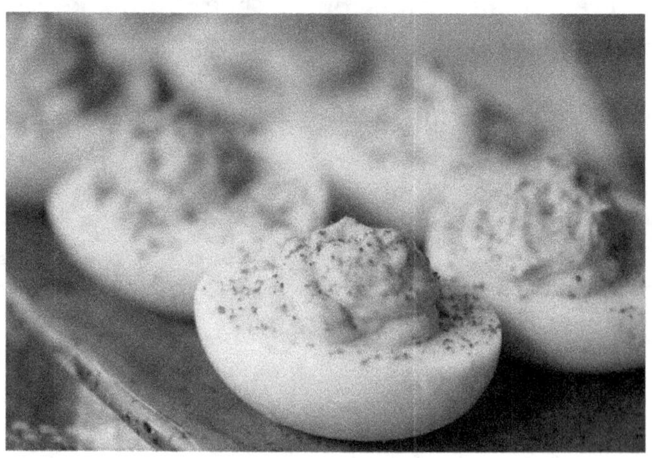

24 servings
Macronutrients: 3 g Protein |7 g Fats |1 g Carb| -0- g Net Carbs

Ingredients:

- 12 large eggs
- 1/2 cup mayonnaise
- 1 tbsp. ground mustard
- 1/4 cup sour cream
- 1 tsp. paprika
- Pinch of:
  - Salt
  - Black pepper

Method:

1. Hard-boil the eggs in 3-4 inches of water. Turn on the stovetop burner to high. After the eggs start to boil; just turn off the heat to the stove. Put a lid on the pan and let it rest for 15 minutes.
2. Drain the eggs and place in an ice bath to chill. Peel and place on a paper towel-lined platter. Slice lengthwise into halves. Remove and mash the yolks.

Mix with the mustard, sour cream, salt, pepper, and mayonnaise.

3. Once it's creamy smooth, scoop it back into the egg halves. Tip: Use a cake decoration bag for a pretty design.

4. Sprinkle with paprika and serve or save for later.

11.8. Desserts

Chocolate Avocado Pudding

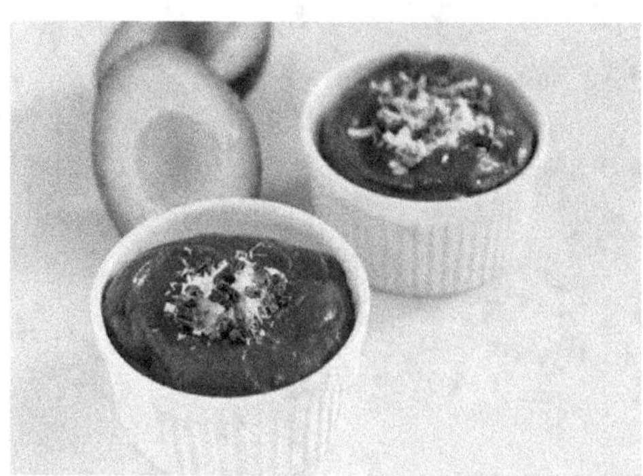

2 servings
Macronutrients: 8 g Protein |27 g Fats| 12 g Carbs| 2 g Net Carbs

Ingredients:
- 2 oz room temperature cream cheese
- 1 ripe med. avocado
- 1 tsp. natural sweetener – swerve
- 1/4 t. vanilla extract
- 4 tbsp. unsweetened cocoa powder
- Pinch of pink salt

Method:
1. Combine the cream cheese with the avocado, sweetener, vanilla, cocoa powder, and salt. Add to a blender or processor.
2. Pulse until creamy smooth.
3. Measure into two fancy dessert dishes and chill for at least 30 minutes.

Chocolate Mousse

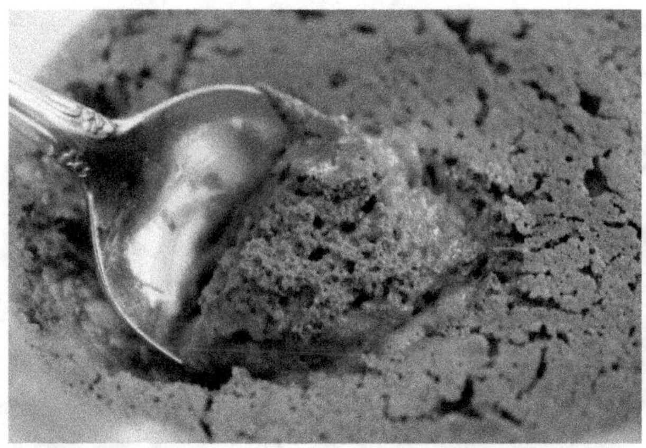

2 servings
Macronutrients: 4 g Protein | 50 g Fats | 5 g Carbs| 4 g Net Carbs

Ingredients:
- 1 1/2 tbsp. heavy whipping cream
- 1 tbsp. of each:
  -Unsweetened cocoa powder
  -Swerve or another natural sweetener
- 4 tbsp. room temperature - of each:
  -Butter
  -Cream Cheese

Method:
1. Chill a bowl and whisk the cream. Store in the fridge.
2. In another dish, use a hand mixer to combine the sweetener, cream cheese, cocoa powder, and butter until well mixed.
3. Take out the refrigerated cream and fold into the chocolate mixture using a rubber scraper.
4. Portion into two dessert dishes and chill for one hour.

Chocolate Shakes

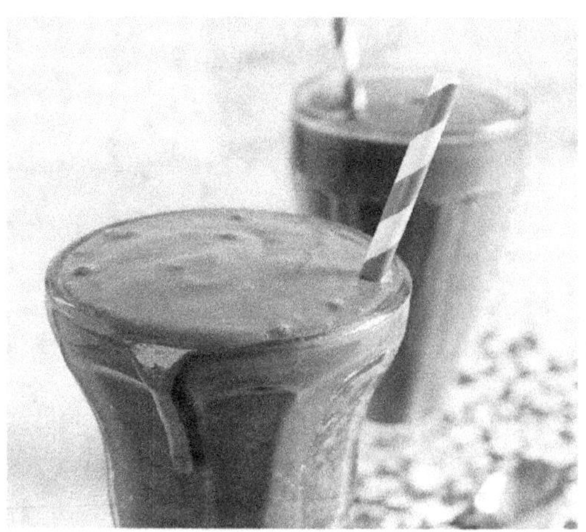

2 servings
Macronutrients: 4 g Protein | 47 g Fats |15 g Carbs| 7 g Net Carbs

Ingredients:
- 4 oz. coconut milk
- 3/4 cup heavy whipping cream
- 1 tbsp. natural sweetener – swerve
- 1/4 tsp. vanilla extract
- 2 tbsp. unsweetened cocoa powder

Method:
1. Empty the cream into a cold metal bowl. Use your hand mixer and cold beaters to form peaks.
2. Slowly add the milk into the cream. Add the rest of the fixings.
3. Stir well and portion into two glasses. Chill in the freezer one hour before serving. Tip: Stir a couple of times if possible.

Crustless Cheesecake Bites

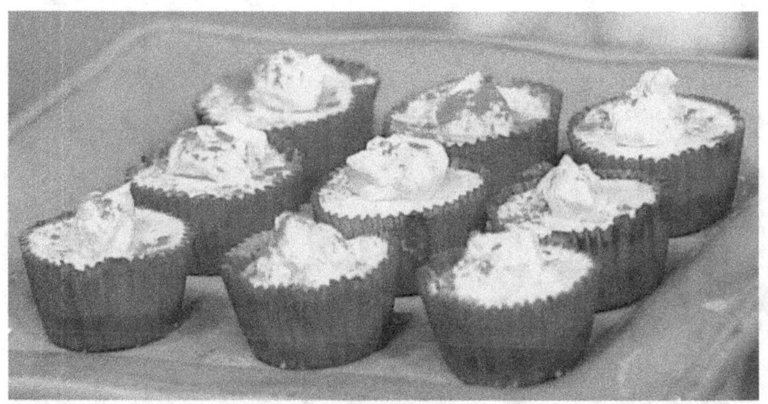

4 servings
Macronutrients: 5 g Protein | 15 g Fats | 2 g Carbs| 2 g Net Carbs

Ingredients:

- 2 large eggs
- 1/4 cup sour cream
- 4 oz. room temperature cream cheese
- 1/4 tsp. vanilla extract
- 1/3 cup natural sweetener – ex. swerve

Method:

1. Warm up the oven temperature to 350°F.
2. Use a hand mixer to combine the fixings.
3. Line a muffin pan with 4 paper or silicone liners.
4. Fill the cups and bake for 30 minutes.
5. After cooling about 3 hours, serve and enjoy.
6. You can save the extras in the freezer for up to 3 months if stored in zip-lock type bags.

Lemon Blueberry Muffins

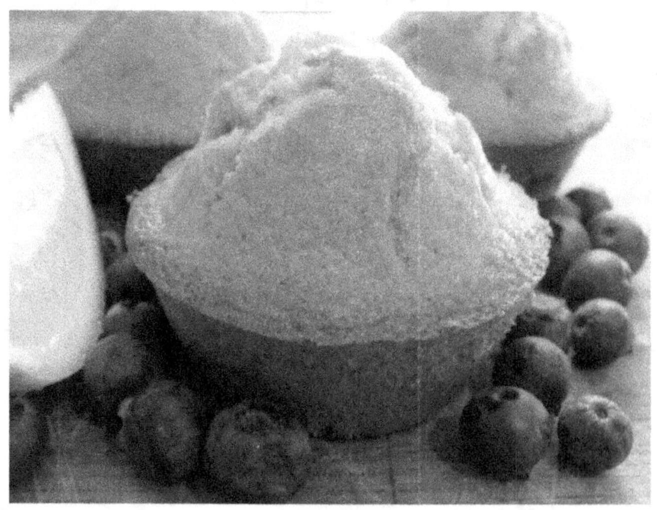

5 servings
Macronutrients: 3 g Protein | 23 g Fats | 6.2 g Carbs| 4.6 g
Net Carbs

Ingredients:
- 1 cup heavy cream
- 2 cups almond flour
- 2 eggs
- 5 tsp. sweetener of choice
- 1/8 cup melted butter
- 1/4 tsp. salt
- 1/2 tsp. of each:
  -Dried lemon zest
  -Lemon extract
  -Baking soda
- 4 oz. blueberries

Method:
1. Warm up the oven to reach 350°F. Place cup liners
   into a 12-count muffin tin.

2. Combine the heavy cream and butter. Crack and stir
    in the eggs one at a time. Mix in the rest of the fixings
    – omitting the berries for now. Stir well.
3. Gently fold in the berries and spoon into the prepared
    cups. Fill halfway.
4. Bake until browned (20 min.).

Lemonade Fat Bombs

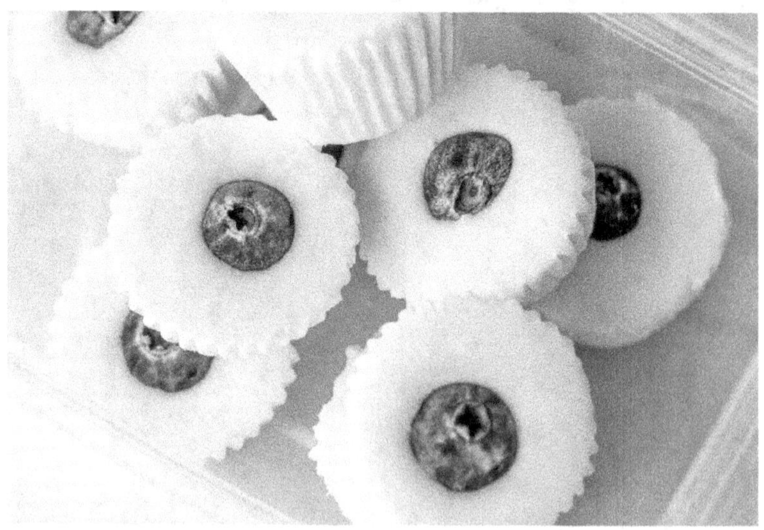

2 servings
Macronutrients: 4 g Protein | 43 g Fats | 8 Carbs| 7 g Net Carbs

Ingredients:
- 4 oz cream cheese
- 2 oz. butter
- 1/2 of a lemon
- 2 t. swerve/2 drops liquid stevia
- Pinch of Pink Himalayan salt

Method:
1. Take the butter and cream cheese out of the fridge and let it become room temperature before using.
2. Zest the lemon and juice it into a small dish.
3. In another container, mix the butter with the cream cheese. Use a hand mixer to combine all of the fixings until well mixed.
4. Spoon the mixture into small molds or cupcake paper liners in a muffin tin pan.

5. Stick the chosen holder in the freezer for two hours. Take them out of the molds and put them in a zipper-top baggie to enjoy any time. Store in the freezer compartment for up to three months.
6. Add a blueberry in the center for a change of pace (0.2 extranet carbs).

NY Cheesecake Cupcakes

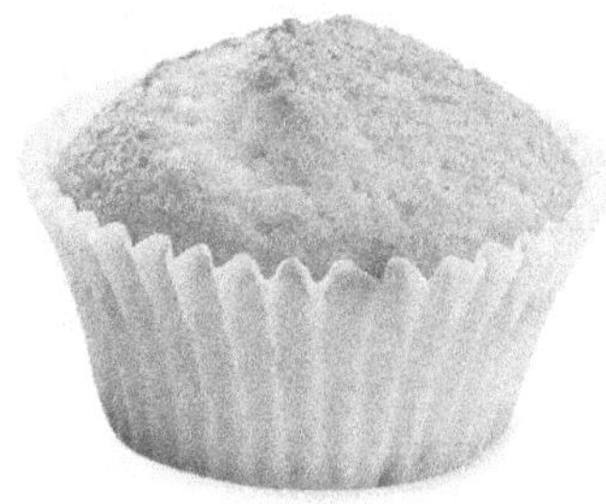

12 servings
Macronutrients: 6.5 g Protein | 26.7 g Fats | 15.5 g Carbs|
14.7 g Net Carbs

Ingredients:
- 2 pkg. (8oz. ea.) cream cheese
- 1/2 cup sour cream
- 5 tbsp. melted butter
- 2/3 cup almond meal
- 3/4 c. swerve or another favorite
- 3 eggs
- 1/4 cup heavy whipping cream
- 2 tbsp of each:
  -Almond flour
  -Water
- 1 1/2 tsp. vanilla extract

Method:
1. Warm up the oven until it reaches 350°F.
2. Prepare a 12-count muffin pan with paper liners.
3. Combine the butter and almond meal and spoon into the liners to form the crust.

4. Stir the sweetener and cream cheese until creamy. Blend in with the water and whipping cream. One at a time, add the eggs, stirring with each one.
5. Next, fold in the flour, sour cream, and extract. Spoon into the liners.
6. Bake for 15-18 minutes. Don't over-cook. The middle will be set when it's done. Cool on the countertop until room temperature. Then, store in the fridge overnight or a minimum of 8 hours.

Peanut Butter & Chocolate Cups

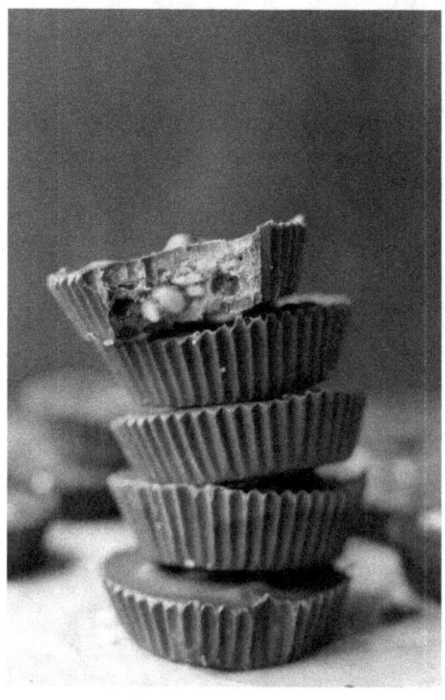

12 servings
Macronutrients: 3.4 g Protein | 26 g Fats | 3.3 g Carbs| 2.2 g
Net Carbs

Ingredients:
- 1 cup coconut oil
- 2 tbsp. heavy cream
- 1/2 cup natural peanut butter or other butter
- 1 tbsp. cocoa powder
- 1/4 tsp. of each:
  - Kosher salt
  - Vanilla extract
- 1 oz. roasted chopped salted peanuts or another favorite keto-friendly nut

Method:

1. Use the low setting on the stovetop to prepare a saucepan with the coconut oil. Once it's hot (3-5 min.), stir in the rest of the fixings.
2. Pour into the silicone muffin molds or use an ice tray. Sprinkle with the nuts and put them on a baking tray.
3. Freeze until it's firm for about one hour. Pop out of the molds and place in an airtight container to enjoy.

Raspberry Fudge

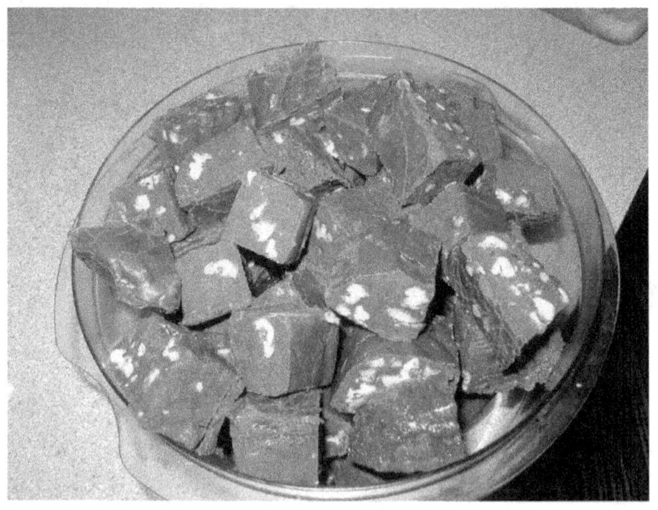

12 servings
Macronutrients: 2.6 g Protein |25.3 g Fats | 5.5 g Carbs| 4.4 g Net Carbs

Ingredients:
- 1 cup butter
- 1 pkg. (8 oz.) cream cheese
- 6 tbsp. unsweetened cocoa powder
- 2 tbsp. heavy cream
- 1/4 cup white sugar substitute
- 2 tsp. vanilla extract
- 1 tsp. raspberry extract
- 1/3 c. chopped walnuts

Method:
1. Take the cream cheese and butter out of the fridge ahead of time until it reaches room temperature.
2. Mix the butter and cream cheese in a large microwavable container using an electric mixer. When smooth, combine with the rest of the fixings and stir until well mixed.

3. Microwave using the high setting for 30 seconds. Blend with the mixer again until smooth.
4. Empty into the prepared pan (1-inch layer). Place a lid on the container. Put it in the fridge to chill for a minimum of two hours.
5. Slice into 12 portions and serve or store.

11.9. Appetizers & Snacks

Cheese Chips & Guacamole

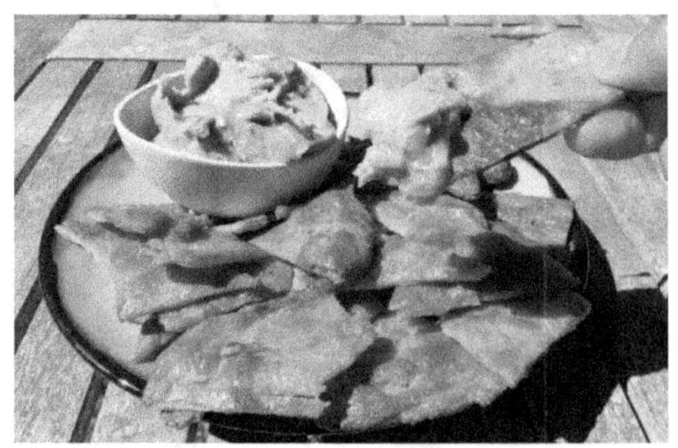

2 servings
Macronutrients: 15 g Protein | 27 g Fats |8 g Carbs| 3 g Net Carbs

Ingredients:
- 1 cup Mexican blend shredded cheese
- Juice of 1/2 of a lime
- 1 mashed avocado
- 2 tbsp. chopped cilantro leaves
- To Taste:
  -Freshly cracked black pepper
  -Pink Himalayan salt
- 1 tsp. diced jalapenos

Method:
1. Warm up the oven until it reaches 350°F. Prepare a baking tin with a sheet of parchment paper. You can also use a silicone baking mat.
2. Create mounds (1/4 cup each) of the cheese on the pan. Leave room between each one and bake for 7 minutes. The centers will be fully melted with browned edges.

3. When done, set on the countertop to cool (5 min.). They will crisp up as they cool.
4. Prepare the Guacamole: Combine the lime juice, avocado, cilantro, salt, pepper, and jalapenos. Mix well and top off with the cheese chips to serve.

Chicken-Pecan Salad & Cucumber Bites

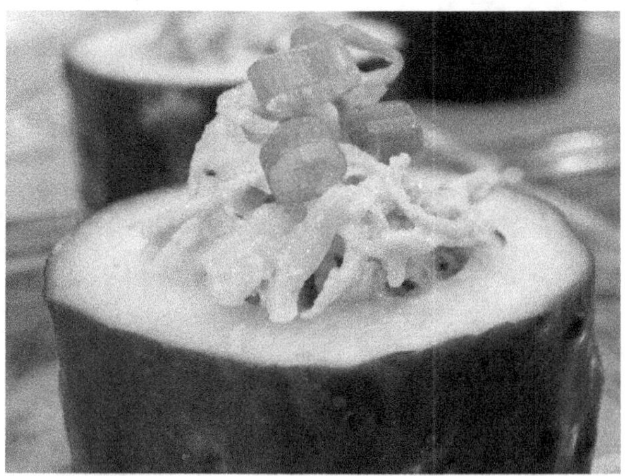

2 servings
Macronutrients: 23 g Protein | 24 g Fats |6 g Carbs| 3 g Net Carbs

Ingredients:
- 2 tbsp. mayonnaise
- 1 cup cooked chicken breast
- 1 cucumber
- 1/4 cup of each:
  -Diced celery
  -Chopped pecans
- Pinch of each:
- To Taste:
  -Freshly cracked black pepper
  -Pink Himalayan salt

Method:
1. Peel (or leave the peel on if desired) and slice the cucumber into 1/4-inch slices. Dice the chicken and celery. Chop the pecans.
2. Combine the pecans, chicken, mayo, and celery in a salad bowl. Sprinkle with the pepper and salt.
3. Lay out the cucumber slices and add a pinch of salt. Layer each one with a spoonful of the chicken salad.

4. Serve.

Crunchy Zucchini Sticks

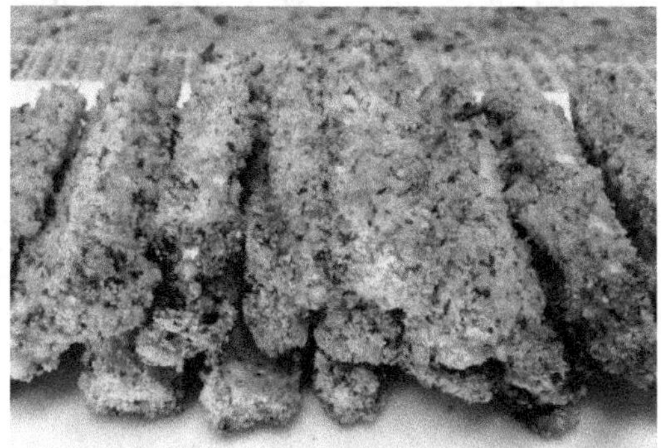

2 servings
Macronutrients: 9 g Protein | 20 g Fats |8 g Carbs| 6 g Net Carbs

Ingredients:
- 2 tbsp. butter
- 2 med. zucchini
- 1/4 cup of each:
  -Crushed pork rinds
  -Parmesan cheese
- 2 garlic cloves
- For drizzling: Olive oil
- To Taste:
  -Freshly cracked black pepper
  -Pink Himalayan salt

Method:
1. Heat up the oven to reach 400°F. Prepare a baking tin with a silicone baking mat or some foil.
2. Slice the zucchini lengthwise and remove the seeds. Slice and arrange them on the baking sheet. Combine the cheese, pork rinds, melted butter, and garlic. Dredge the slices through the mixture. Give it a shake of pepper and salt.

3. Drizzle with the oil and bake 20 minutes or until it's crunchy like you like it.
4. Warm up the oven broiler and cook 3-5 minutes before serving.

Smoked Salmon & Cream Cheese Roll-Ups

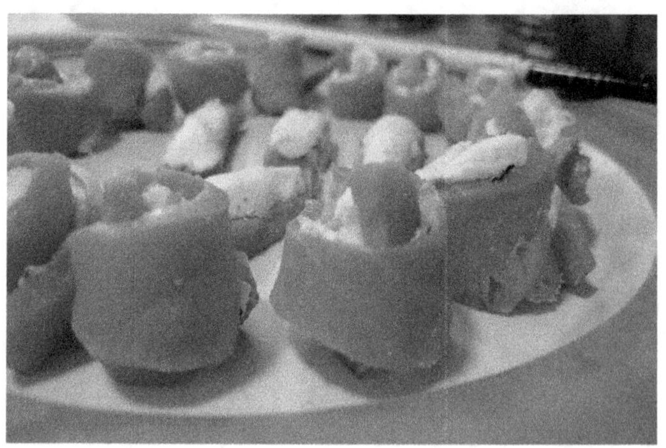

2 servings
Macronutrients: 14 g Protein | 22 g Fats |4 g Carbs| 3 g Net Carbs

Ingredients:
- 2 tbsp chopped scallions – green and white parts
- 1 tsp. of each:
  -Dijon mustard
  -Grated lemon zest
- 4 oz. each:
  -Room temperature cream cheese
  -Cold smoked salmon – 12 slices
- To Taste:
  -Freshly cracked black pepper
  -Pink Himalayan salt

Method:
1. Mix the lemon zest, cream cheese, scallions, and mustard using a blender or food processor. Flavor with the pepper and salt. Mix until creamy smooth.
2. Spread the cheese mix on both sides of the salmon and roll. Arrange with the seam-side down on a platter.

3. Cover with plastic and place in the fridge until ready
    to eat. They will remain fresh for about 3 days.

Chapter 12: Your 14-Day Meal Plan

You should have a good understanding of how to prepare your own meal plan after you enjoy the one that is set up for 14 days. Each one of the days has a main meal for breakfast, a snack, lunch, dinner, and a dessert. Each one is close to the 20 grams for optimal weight loss. Remember, you have some 'wiggle' room here, depending on how many extra carbs you want to add to your daily tally.

I have also provided a few extra tips when you start flying solo.

Let's Begin!

DAY 1:

1. Breakfast: Bacon – Spinach - Avocado & Egg: 4 g
2. Snack: Cheese Chips & Guacamole: 3 g
3. Lunch: Broccoli & Cheese Soup: 3 g
    Keto Bread: 2 g
    Vegetarian Deviled Eggs: 0 g
4. Dinner: Buffalo Chicken Casserole: 5.1 g
    Keto Bread: 2 g
5. Dessert: Chocolate Avocado Pudding: 2 g

Totals of Net Carbs – Day 1: 21.1 g

DAY 2:

1. Breakfast: BLT Breakfast Salad: 4 g
2. Snack: Smoked Salmon & Cream Cheese Roll-Ups – No-Cook: 3 g
3. Lunch: Pizza Bites: 2.8 g
    Broccoli – 1/2 cup fresh broccoli: 4.04 g
4. Dinner: Bun-Less Bacon Burgers: 2.2 g
    Cheese Chips & Guacamole: 3 g
5. Dessert: Crustless Cheesecake Bites: 2 g

Totals of Net Carbs – Day 2: 21.04 g

DAY 3:

1. Breakfast: Baked Eggs in Avocado: 2 g
2. Snack or with Lunch: Cheese Chips & Guacamole: 3 g
3. Lunch: Carnitas - Crockpot: 4 g
4. Dinner: Fried Pork Chops: 4.2 g
   Buttery Mushrooms - Slow Cooked: 3 g
5. Dessert: Chocolate Mousse: 4 g

Totals of Net Carbs – Day 3: 20.2 g

DAY 4:

1. Breakfast: Brussels Sprouts, Eggs & Bacon for Brunch: 7 g
2. Snack: Vegetarian Deviled Eggs: 0 g
3. Lunch: Alfredo Pizza: 2.8 g
4. Dinner: Beef Short Ribs: 2.5 g
   Baked Zucchini Gratin: 3 g
5. Dessert: Lemon Blueberry Muffins: 4.6 g

Totals of Net Carbs – Day 4: 19.9 g

DAY 5:

1. Breakfast: Cheesy Egg & Spinach Nest: 4 g
2. Snack: Chicken-Pecan Salad & Cucumber Bites – No Cook: 3 g
3. Lunch: Pork Kabobs: 3.3 g
   Cheese Chips & Guacamole: 3 g
4. Dinner: Chuck Steak – Slow Cooker: 2.9 g
   Buttery Mushrooms - Slow Cooked: 3 g
1. Dessert: Peanut Butter & Chocolate Cups: 2.2 g

Totals of Net Carbs – Day 5: 21.4 g

DAY 6:

1. Breakfast: Coconut Flour – Cream Cheese Pancakes: 4 g
2. Snack: Vegetarian Deviled Eggs: 0 g

3. Lunch: Bacon Stir Fry for Brunch: 8 g
4. Dinner: Coconut Shrimp: 1.1 g
   Salmon & Caesar Salad: 2 g
5. Dessert: Raspberry Fudge: 4.4 g

Totals of Net Carbs – Day 6: 19.5 g

DAY 7:

1. Breakfast: Cheesy Muffins: 4.3 g
2. Snack or part of Lunch Crunchy Zucchini Sticks: 6 g
3. Lunch: Chicken Salad: 8 g
4. Dinner: Feta-Stuffed Burgers: 1 g
5. Dessert: Raspberry Fudge: 4.4 g

Totals of Net Carbs – Day 7: 23.7 g

DAY 8:

2. Breakfast: Kale – Avocado & Egg Skillet: 6 g
3. Snack or with Lunch: Cheese Chips & Guacamole: 3 g
4. Lunch: Chopped Greek Salad: 2 g
5. Dinner: Cheesy Steak: 9.6 g
   Vegetarian Deviled Egg: 0 g
6. Dessert: Peanut Butter & Chocolate Cups: 2.2 g

Totals of Net Carbs – Day 8: 22.8 g

DAY 9:

1. Breakfast: Perfect Scrambled Eggs: 1 g
2. Snack: Baked Zucchini Gratin: 3 g
3. Lunch: Shrimp & Avocado Salad: 3 g
4. Dinner: Fried Pork Chops: 4.2 g
   Tomato – Avocado & Cucumber Salad: 6 g
5. Dessert: Chocolate Shakes: 7 g

Totals of Net Carbs – Day 9: 24.2 g

DAY 10:

1. Breakfast: Cheesy Muffins: 4.3 g
2. Snack: Crustless Cheesecake Bites: 2 g
3. Lunch: Tomato – Avocado & Cucumber Salad: 6 g
   Snack: Vegetarian Deviled Eggs: 0 g
4. Dinner: Garlic Parmesan Wings: 5.3 g
   Broccoli & Cheese Soup: 3 g
5. Dessert: Chocolate Avocado Pudding: 2 g

Totals of Net Carbs – Day 10: 22.6 g

DAY 11:

1. Breakfast: Coconut Flour – Cream Cheese Pancakes: 4 g
2. Snack: Cheese Chips & Guacamole: 3 g
3. Lunch: Alfredo Pizza: 2.8 g
   Chopped Greek Salad: 2 g
4. Dinner: Meatballs in the Crock: 3.7 g
   Chopped Greek Salad: 2 g
5. Dessert: Chocolate Mousse: 4 g

Totals of Net Carbs – Day 11: 21.5 g

DAY 12:

1. Breakfast: Cheesy Egg & Spinach Nest: 4 g
2. Snack: Raspberry Fudge: 4.4 g
3. Lunch: Dinner: Crockpot Chicken Chowder: 7.5 g
4. Dinner: Beef Short Ribs: 2.5 g
5. Dessert: Lemon Blueberry Muffins: 4.6 g

Totals of Net Carbs – Day 12: 23 g

DAY 13:

1. Breakfast: BLT Breakfast Salad: 4 g
2. Snack: Smoked Salmon & Cream Cheese Roll-Ups – No-Cook: 3 g
3. Lunch: Carnitas - Crockpot: 4 g

4. Dinner: Steak Pinwheels: 2.1 g
   Broccoli & Cheese Soup: 3 g
5. Dessert: Chocolate Avocado Pudding: 2 g

Totals of Net Carbs – Day 13: 18.1 g

Day 14:

1. Breakfast: Baked Eggs in Avocado: 2 g
2. Snack: Raspberry Fudge: 4.4 g
3. Lunch: Cucumber Sandwich: 12.6 g
4. Dinner: Pork Kabobs: 3.3 g
5. Dessert: Crustless Cheesecake Bites: 2 g

Totals of Net Carbs – Day 14: 24.3

Planning Your Menu

Now that you know what foods to eat on the keto diet, it's time to start putting a meal plan together. First, take a look at the list of foods allowed on a diet and choose foods you actually enjoy. There is no point in trying to follow a diet that is full of things you hate.

Carve out some time on a Sunday to plan your meals. This may seem burdensome at first, but planning ahead is the best way to ensure success.

Next start building meals around three main items: protein, fat, and a vegetable. This will ensure you are getting balanced meals, helping you stay satisfied. Plan for three meals a day and a few snacks. You may find that because keto suppresses your appetite after a few weeks, you might not need to eat that often.

Here are some examples of how to build meals using that pattern:

Breakfast: Ham and cheese omelet with spinach

Protein: Eggs, Ham, or Cheese

Fat: Butter

Vegetable: Spinach

Lunch: Bun-less hamburger

Protein: Hamburger Patty

Fat: Avocado

Vegetables: Lettuce, tomato, and pickles

Dinner: Chicken and vegetables

Protein: Chicken

Fat: Butter - for veggies

Vegetables: A variety of veggies such as broccoli, cauliflower, etc.

In Closing: Choose recipes that are quick and easy to make or can be prepared ahead of time for busy nights. Start keeping a notebook with a list of recipes you enjoy, so you don't need to search for new ideas every time. Also, plan for some leftovers for lunches or snacks, so you don't have to cook for every single meal.

Now you have 14 days of meals and snacks ready to go, you won't need to scramble to figure out what to eat at the last minute. With all of the recipes listed having detailed nutritional counts, you won't leave the state of 'ketosis' until you are ready. Enjoy the ketogenic recipes and remain healthy.

Conclusion

I hope you enjoyed each page-turning chapter of the *Ketogenic Diet: The Complete Guide to Healthy Weight Loss*. I hope as you read through your personal copy, that it provided you with all of the tools you need to achieve your goals of controlling your weight and enjoying a healthier lifestyle.

The next step is to recall the essential foods along with the 'not so good' items on the ketogenic diet plan. Compile a shopping list of all of the things you want to prepare for a couple of days. All of the nutritional counts are provided within each of the recipes, so just stay within the carbohydrate limitations of your chosen type of plan.

Once your meal plan is complete make a list of ingredients that you will need and head for the store. Be sure not to go hungry, or you will end up with a ton of things that don't match your plan. The key to sticking with your meal plan is having the right items on hand when you need them. You need to make it as easy as possible to reach for the right things.

If you have tons of items in your pantry that are not allowed on your diet, it will be pretty challenging to stick with it, particularly the first week or so when you are still adjusting to the techniques, and the appetite suppression part hasn't kicked in yet. Consider hiding foods that are triggers for you to overeat or give them to a friend.

If possible, once you return from the store spend a little time cooking and prepping for the week. Grill some chicken or steak for easy meals, make enough to last for three days, so you don't have to cook again until Wednesday. Use the protein to top salads or add a side of broccoli or cauliflower for a full meal. Chop some veggies or pre-portion a few nuts for snacks.

Planning meals a week at a time is the best way to be sure you stay on track. The important thing is to remain consistent. Meal planning and prepping can be a little time-consuming. However, without planning ahead and having the items you need on hand, it can be tempting to slip into old habits.

Consider using one of the intermittent fasting techniques to boost your ketosis along. After all, you are in the phase of ketosis as you sleep. Remain strong-minded and stick to your goals during your transition to ketosis. Each of the recipes in this diet plan has been researched with your goals in mind. Follow the directions and recipe preparation methods. Before long, you will be exercising and cooking much healthier meals for you and your family. Set the goals and know how your body will react to the changes it will make during the process.

You are human and sometimes will slip with a hot fudge sundae or another delicious 'sugary' treat. If you do, just get back on the right path and let it go. Life happens; you might just need a little longer to get the diet into motion while you lose those cravings. You will be too full to worry about consuming the wasted calories for one little treat. Move forward; tomorrow is a fresh day.

After you have started losing your weight, it's essential to have a bit of fun. However, you should be sure it is not a food-related treat unless it's keto-friendly. Buy a new outfit to show off your weight loss. Take the family for an evening on-the-town. You deserve it.

Finally, if you found this book useful in any way, a review on Amazon is always appreciated!

Click here to leave a review on Amazon!

https://www.amazon.es/dp/1798540045